The Pink Salt Trick Weight Loss Recipe Book & Diet Guide

A Complete Pink Salt Cookbook for Fat Burn, Detox, Craving Control, Hormone Reset & Natural Weight Loss Without Pills

Jerry A. Hannon

Contents

Introduction

This Isn't Just About Salt—It's About Taking Your Power Back

There's a moment—quiet, subtle, and usually in the mirror—when you realize something has to change. Not in a dramatic, rock-bottom way. Just a whisper. A tightening waistband that didn't used to be tight. The fog in your head that no amount of coffee can lift. The afternoon energy crash that seems to hit harder every day. The growing list of foods your body no longer "tolerates." And worst of all, the nagging fear that this is your new normal.

But what if that whisper isn't a warning… it's an invitation?

What if the solution isn't another restrictive diet or complicated routine, but a **ritual**—a small, grounded, consistent act that works with your body instead of against it?

What if the answer has been hiding in something as elemental as **salt**?

Yes—salt. But not the kind your doctor warned you about. Not the white, lifeless grains dumped into processed foods. This is *Himalayan pink salt*—raw, mineral-rich, and ancient. The kind of salt that still remembers oceans before they became deserts. The kind of salt that doesn't just flavor your food but fuels your cells, stabilizes your hormones, sharpens your mind, and calms your nervous system.

And when taken intentionally—as a **simple morning drink**—this salt can help you reclaim more than just your waistline. It can help you reclaim your rhythm.

What This Book Is—and What It Is Not

This is not a weight loss gimmick wrapped in a pretty cover.
This is not a "new diet" dressed in a different outfit.
This is not a plan that asks you to count, restrict, punish, or obsess.

This book is a **biological reboot**, rooted in simplicity and truth. It's about **re-educating your body and mind** through one deceptively small practice: a 5-minute morning ritual involving water, pink salt, and conscious intention.

It's also a complete, reader-friendly **cookbook**, a **craving-control toolkit**, and a **metabolism reset protocol** for women and men who are sick of being told they're "lazy" or "undisciplined." You'll find **101 recipes, science-backed explanations**, and a **21-day plan** to help you shift not just your weight—but your mindset, energy, and self-trust.

And yes, it works without pills, powders, or pricey supplements.

Why This Works When Everything Else Hasn't

Because this isn't about **manipulating your body**—it's about **listening to it.**

When your body is out of rhythm, it speaks in symptoms: stubborn fat, fatigue, cravings, anxiety, bloating, and brain fog. These aren't failures. They're signals.

The pink salt ritual helps your body remember what it already knows: how to **burn fat naturally**, how to **stabilize blood sugar**, how to **balance your hormones**, and how to **hydrate on a cellular level**.

It clears the fog, quiets the chaos, and restores the conditions your metabolism needs to function—not fight.

This book shows you how.

The Real Weight You're Losing

If you've been stuck in a cycle of start-and-stop wellness attempts, you're not alone. What most people want isn't just to "lose weight"—it's to **feel light again**. In their body. In their skin. In their mind.

They want to wake up with clarity. To eat without shame. To move without pain. To wear clothes without second-guessing. To go through the day without dragging.

They want peace. Power. **Freedom.**

That's what this book is really about.

How to Use This Book

You don't need to read it all at once. Start with the chapter that speaks to where you are. If you're curious about the pink salt drink, jump into the ritual. If you're tired of conflicting advice, skip to the hormone and craving chapters. If you're ready for full transformation, go all in with the 21-Day Pink Salt Reset.

Whatever pace you choose, **you will not get overwhelmed**. There are no tables. No gimmicks. No technical jargon. Just **honest, powerful, and practical guidance** written for humans—with zero fluff and no sugar-coating.

This is a book designed to fit real life.
To meet you where you are.
And to walk with you—step by step—back to balance.

One Small Ritual. One Big Return.

So if you're tired of starting over, of feeling like your body is broken, of spending money on supplements and solutions that overpromise and underdeliver…

Consider this your moment.

Your pink salt.
Your glass of water.
Your 5-minute reset.

And a book that will remind you—**you were never actually that far off track.**

Let's begin.

Chapter 1

The Pink Salt Trick—What It Is & Why It Works

She stood in front of her mirror, half-awake, still wrapped in a faded robe that had known too many Monday mornings. Her hand clutched a warm glass of water tinged with a soft pink hue—Himalayan salt dissolved like a secret. It wasn't a diet. It wasn't a fast. It was something quieter, more intuitive. And yet, it was the one thing that finally shifted everything.

Welcome to the ritual that's transforming women's mornings across the world—one pinch of pink salt at a time.

What Makes Pink Salt So Unique?

(Mineral Profile + Cellular Hydration)

At a glance, pink Himalayan salt looks like just another gourmet addition to a trendy kitchen. But at a biological level, it's a mineral powerhouse sourced from ancient seabeds beneath the Himalayan mountains—untouched by modern pollution, rich in over **84 trace minerals**. These include:

- **Magnesium**, essential for metabolic regulation and muscle relaxation

- **Potassium**, which balances fluid levels and prevents bloating
- **Calcium**, necessary for nerve signaling and fat metabolism
- **Sodium**, the misunderstood mineral that fuels cellular function
- **Iron**, giving the salt its iconic pink hue—and aiding oxygen transport
- **Zinc, iodine, selenium**, and other key electrolytes that support immunity, thyroid balance, and hormone regulation

These minerals aren't isolated. They exist in an ionic state that mirrors the **electrolyte composition of your blood plasma**, making pink salt incredibly bioavailable—your cells recognize it and absorb it efficiently. That's why drinking pink salt first thing in the morning doesn't just hydrate—it *reboots* your cellular function.

Think of it as sending your body the correct passcode to unlock its natural systems again—digestion, metabolism, and energy regulation—all before your first bite of food.

The Morning Pink Salt Drink: How It Became Viral

In a world flooded with weight-loss gimmicks, TikTok influencers and wellness coaches began whispering about an ancient ritual: a teaspoon of pink Himalayan salt in warm water upon waking. But this wasn't new. Ayurvedic healers, traditional Chinese medicine practitioners, and even Native American herbalists have long known the connection between mineral balance and morning detox.

So why did it suddenly catch fire online?

Because women began reporting real, tangible results—often within days:

- A flatter belly without changing what they ate
- Fewer cravings for sugar and carbs
- Clearer skin and better digestion
- Consistent energy without coffee crashes
- Deep, uninterrupted sleep

The virality wasn't manufactured—it was **earned by results.** And for women burned by years of restrictive diets and supplement overkill, this one simple shift felt like relief wrapped in ritual.

How It Works: Craving Control, Hydration & Hormonal Signaling

1. Craving Control

Cravings, particularly for sugar and refined carbs, often stem not from hunger but from **mineral deficiency and blood sugar instability**. Pink salt replenishes sodium, magnesium, and potassium, which calm erratic brain signals that trigger cravings.

Sodium supports adrenal function, which stabilizes **blood glucose response**—making it less likely that you'll experience the "crash" that causes a mid-morning pastry run.

2. Hydration That Reaches Your Cells

Plain water often doesn't hydrate as well as you think. Without minerals, water may pass through the digestive system without being absorbed—leaving cells still thirsty.

Pink salt turns your water into a natural electrolyte drink, improving **osmotic balance**. This means your cells pull in water efficiently, reducing signs of dehydration such as fatigue, dizziness, sugar cravings, and headaches.

3. Hormonal Signaling Reset

Hormones are chemical messengers, and their accuracy depends on having the correct mineral environment. Sodium and magnesium directly affect the **HPA axis**—your body's stress-response system involving the hypothalamus, pituitary, and adrenal glands.

By restoring these minerals in the morning, you:

- Calm cortisol spikes that lead to belly fat
- Reboot insulin sensitivity, helping with fat metabolism
- Support thyroid hormone conversion, improving energy and mood

This is not just hydration—it's **cellular communication therapy**.

Why This Trick Works Without Dieting, Fasting, or Pills

For most women, the problem isn't a lack of willpower—it's a body in **survival mode.**

Decades of yo-yo dieting, low-salt paranoia, and caffeine dependence have created a population of women living with

- Burned-out adrenals
- Chronically elevated cortisol
- Water retention disguised as weight gain
- Constant sugar cravings from blood sugar crashes
- Sluggish digestion and slowed thyroid output

The Pink Salt Trick gently reverses all of that—without requiring deprivation.

Because it addresses **root causes**, not symptoms.

- No calorie tracking
- No app obsession
- No synthetic pills
- No crash diets

It's not a fix you *force* on your body—it's a rhythm your body *remembers.*

The Daily Energy Reset & The Role of Adrenal Balance

Your adrenal glands—those tiny triangle-shaped powerhouses sitting atop your kidneys—are the unsung heroes of your metabolism and mood. They produce cortisol and aldosterone, two hormones that regulate:

- Blood pressure
- Fat storage and energy usage
- Fluid retention and salt balance
- Wake-sleep cycles and alertness

When you wake up depleted, your adrenals often overcompensate—pumping out cortisol to "wake you up," which leads to a chain reaction: hunger, anxiety, energy crashes, and eventually fat storage.

Pink salt supports the **production of aldosterone**, the hormone responsible for **electrolyte balance and blood volume.** When aldosterone is in balance, your body stops hoarding water weight, your energy steadies, and cortisol can finally lower.

Drinking a warm pink salt tonic upon waking tells your adrenals: *"We're safe. You can relax. We have the minerals we need. Let's burn fat and not crash today."*

It's like giving your hormonal orchestra its tuning fork—everything comes back in sync.

A Ritual of Reclamation

For too long, women have been told that weight loss must be hard. That it must involve punishment, hunger, guilt, or control. But what if all that noise has just been drowning out something much simpler?

The Pink Salt Trick isn't about chasing perfection. It's about giving your body the **raw materials it needs** to remember how to function.

It's not magic. It's **mineral logic**.

And in the next chapter, we'll explore how this logic rewrites everything the diet industry has ignored—especially when it comes to hormones, fat storage, and metabolic health.

But first—tomorrow morning, pour yourself a glass of warm water. Stir in a pinch of pink salt. Sit still. Breathe. Sip. Reconnect.

Your body's been waiting for this.

Chapter 2

Fat, Hormones & The Metabolism Reset

If you've ever felt like your body is fighting against you no matter how little you eat or how often you work out, you're not crazy—and you're not alone.

The truth is, weight loss isn't just about calories. It never was. The real game-changer—the lever that quietly controls fat storage, hunger, cravings, and energy—comes down to something deeper: **hormones.**

In this chapter, we're going to unravel why most mainstream weight loss advice is outdated, how pink salt plays a unique role in supporting your hormones, and what it takes to truly reset your metabolism from the inside out.

Because the reason you're tired, bloated, foggy, and stuck has little to do with willpower—and everything to do with what your hormones are whispering beneath the surface.

Why Most Weight Loss Advice Ignores Your Hormones

Open any magazine or scroll through your social feed, and you'll see the same advice repeated like a broken record:

Eat less. Move more. Cut carbs. Count calories. Fast until noon. Take this pill. Avoid salt.

It's the same old formula: Restrict. Burn. Repeat.

But here's what most of those "experts" won't tell you—**your body doesn't burn fat just because you're hungry or sweating.** Your body burns fat when your hormones say it's *safe* to do so.

Let that sink in:

> Fat loss is not a math problem—it's a metabolic permission slip.

And that permission slip is written by your **endocrine system**—the network of glands that release hormones like cortisol, insulin, leptin, ghrelin, thyroid hormones, and estrogen. When these are imbalanced, your body clings to fat, regardless of how little you eat.

Here's where it gets more personal: for most women, especially over 30, **hormonal shifts become the hidden cause of stubborn weight, water retention, brain fog, and fatigue.**

If you've ever felt like the more you restrict, the worse your energy and metabolism get, you're likely caught in the hormone trap. And it's not your fault.

The Pink Salt Trick's Role in Balancing Cortisol, Insulin & Leptin

So how does pink salt—a natural, mineral-rich crystal—play into something as complex as hormone regulation?

Let's break down the three major hormonal players when it comes to weight:

1. Cortisol—The Stress Hormone That Stores Fat

Cortisol gets a bad rap, but it's vital for waking up, energy production, and inflammation control. The issue is **chronic stress**—emotional, physical, and metabolic—keeps cortisol elevated, especially in the morning. High cortisol triggers fat storage (especially belly fat), sugar cravings, and muscle breakdown.

Pink salt helps here in three key ways:

- It supports the **adrenal glands**, which produce cortisol. When your body senses it has enough sodium, it doesn't panic and overproduce stress hormones.
- It **replenishes electrolytes** lost through stress and sleep, helping calm the nervous system.
- It contributes to **hydration and blood pressure regulation**, which lowers the stress load on your cardiovascular system.

In short, a pinch of pink salt in warm water helps signal, "We're *safe." You don't need to hoard fat today."*

2. Insulin—The Gatekeeper of Fat Storage

Insulin's job is to move sugar from your blood into your cells. When you eat too often, consume too much sugar, or experience chronic stress, your body produces more and more insulin—until your cells stop responding.

This condition, called **insulin resistance**, is a precursor to diabetes, belly fat, fatigue, and cravings.

Pink salt's role?

- It helps stabilize **blood sugar spikes** by supporting adrenal and electrolyte balance.
- Minerals like magnesium, chromium, and zinc (found in trace amounts in pink salt) improve **insulin sensitivity**.
- When consumed in the morning before food, it prepares your body to **respond more efficiently** to your first meal—resulting in less insulin output.

This is the difference between burning fat and storing it.

3. Leptin—The Satiety Switch

Leptin is the hormone that tells your brain you're full. But here's the twist: when you gain weight or become inflamed, **leptin resistance** sets in. Your brain stops "hearing" the leptin signals, so you stay hungry, even when your body has enough stored fat.

This is one of the cruelest cycles women fall into: eating less, still feeling hungry, storing fat, and never feeling satisfied.

Pink salt helps by reducing **inflammation** (which improves leptin sensitivity) and by **re-regulating circadian hormones** when used in a morning hydration ritual.

Understanding Metabolic Slowdown & How to Reverse It

Let's talk about your metabolism—not as a number, but as a living, adaptive system.

Your metabolism slows down not just because of age, but because of stress, under-eating, mineral deficiency, and sleep disruption. These send a message to your body: *"Conserve energy. Store fat. Don't risk burning fuel."*

This is what happens when you diet too long or fast too harshly. Your thyroid takes a hit. Your body temperature drops. Your hair thins. Your digestion weakens. Your periods get irregular.

You haven't failed. **Your body is protecting you.**

So how do you reverse it?

By restoring the building blocks your metabolism needs to trust you again:

- **Sodium** to signal safety and fuel adrenal recovery
- **Magnesium** to support cellular energy production (ATP)
- **Potassium and calcium** help regulate insulin and leptin sensitivity
- **Hydration** to improve cellular communication and reduce inflammation

Pink salt provides this base. Not in huge doses—but in precise, consistent morning signals that say:
"It's safe to burn energy now. We're not in a famine. You can let go."

How Mineral Balance Unlocks Fat Burn Without Calorie Tracking

If you've spent years counting every bite, obsessively logging food, and micromanaging meals, this may sound like a fairy tale—but it's physiology.

Fat burning doesn't start in your food journal. It starts in your **mineral balance.**

Here's why:

- Minerals like **magnesium and sodium** regulate mitochondrial function—the little engines in your cells that burn fat.
- Low sodium levels cause **aldosterone spikes**, leading to water retention, bloating, and metabolic slowdown.
- When you're deficient in electrolytes, you crave sugar—not because you need sugar, but because your body is desperate for energy in *any* form.

Fixing this starts with restoring the minerals most women are lacking. The beauty of pink salt is that it's naturally balanced—it doesn't overload one mineral while depleting another.

You begin to feel a shift:

- Steady energy

- No need to snack constantly
- Hunger that's rooted in **real need**, not chaos
- A flatter belly not from starvation—but from balance

You eat intuitively. Move naturally. And your body starts responding the way you always wanted it to.

Hidden Causes of Belly Fat: Water Retention vs. Fat Storage

This might be the most important thing you learn in this chapter:

Not all belly bulge is fat.

In fact, for many women, what they think is "stubborn fat" is actually **mineral imbalance-induced water retention**, combined with chronic inflammation and digestive sluggishness.

Pink salt addresses all three:

1. **Water Retention—**Salt isn't the enemy. It's the imbalance of sodium *without* potassium or hydration that leads to bloating. Pink salt corrects that ratio.
2. Inflammation—The minerals in pink salt help reduce systemic inflammation, a root cause of insulin resistance and leptin confusion.
3. **Digestive Sluggishness—**Salt stimulates **stomach acid production**, improving digestion and reducing bloat that mimics fat gain.

When you reset this foundation, the scale might not immediately drop—but your jeans will fit differently. Your energy will feel different. Your reflection will soften and lift.

Because you're not just losing weight.
You're shedding what your body no longer needs to hold onto.

You're Not Broken. You're Underfed, Undermineralized & Misled

Let's say it clearly: your body hasn't failed you. It's been trying to protect you.

But it was never designed to thrive on:

- Coffee instead of breakfast
- 1,000-calorie diets
- Salt-free "clean eating"
- 12-step fasting plans
- Stress with no recovery

The Pink Salt Trick isn't a trick at all. It's a **return to physiological sanity**—giving your hormones the mineral inputs they've been screaming for, quietly and consistently.

It's not just about looking better. It's about **feeling like yourself again.**

And in the next chapter, we'll break one of the most dangerous cycles women are stuck in: cravings, bloat, and emotional eating.

And how pink salt offers a radical reset—starting not in your diet, but in your brain.

Because the shift you're seeking doesn't come from another rule. It comes from *reclaiming* your rhythm.

Chapter 3

Breaking the Cycle—Cravings, Bloat & Emotional Eating

You don't binge on sugar because you're weak.
You don't feel bloated every afternoon because your body is broken.
You don't reach for food when you're tired, sad, anxious, or overwhelmed because you "lack discipline."

You do it because your body is whispering for help—and no one taught you how to listen.

In this chapter, we're going to dismantle one of the most painful and personal cycles millions of women live through daily: the emotional and biological feedback loop that keeps you stuck between cravings, bloating, guilt, and the shame of not being able to stop.

But there is a way out.

And it doesn't start with willpower.
It starts with salt.

How Pink Salt Helps Curb Sugar Cravings & Binge Triggers

Let's begin with something radical: **cravings are not the enemy.**

Cravings are communication. They're your body's way of signaling a need—often for energy, minerals, safety, or comfort. But because we've been taught to fear them or fight them, we miss the message and respond with restriction or shame.

And nothing intensifies a craving faster than **mineral deficiency.**

Here's why pink salt helps:

- **Sodium** is required for blood sugar regulation and adrenal function. When you're low, your body demands fast fuel—*aka* sugar.
- **Magnesium** (naturally found in pink salt in trace amounts) plays a key role in serotonin production, mood stability, and reducing PMS-triggered cravings.
- **Hydration with minerals** reduces the stress load on your nervous system, which lessens emotional hunger cues.

When you start your day with the Pink Salt Morning Drink, you preemptively fill the gaps that cause afternoon breakdowns. You silence the scream before it starts.

Over time, your brain begins to trust that energy is available, minerals are present, and survival is not in question.
The urgency behind cravings fades.
The grip around sugar softens.

You're not resisting.
You're simply not desperate anymore.

Salt's Role in Gut-Brain Signaling & Mood Stabilization

The gut isn't just your digestion center—it's your second brain.

Nearly 90% of your body's **serotonin**, the "feel-good" hormone, is produced in the gut. And this production is deeply influenced by your gut lining, microbiome health, hydration status, and **mineral composition.**

So when digestion slows down, when bloating increases, when your belly feels inflamed and heavy—it affects your mood. Not metaphorically. *Chemically.*

Pink salt supports this gut-brain connection in several profound ways:

1. **Increased Stomach Acid Production**—Low stomach acid is a hidden epidemic, especially among women who diet. It leads to poor digestion, nutrient malabsorption, and gas. Pink salt stimulates the vagus nerve and gastric acid production, improving digestion at the root.

2. **Improved Gut Motility**—Sodium helps regulate nerve signals that stimulate smooth muscle contraction in the intestines, helping move food (and waste) more efficiently. Less stagnation = less bloating.

3. **Neurotransmitter Support**— Minerals like magnesium, potassium, and sodium support **nervous system balance,**

helping regulate the HPA axis (the system that controls your stress response).

With just one small ritual, you're creating a ripple effect:
Better digestion → Better mood → Fewer cravings → Clearer thoughts → Lighter body.

It's not a cleanse. It's a **neural reset.**

Bloating vs. Fat: What Most Women Are Really Struggling With

You step on the scale, and it's up three pounds overnight. Your jeans feel tight. Your stomach looks swollen by evening.

You think, "I've *gained fat.*"

But 9 out of 10 times, that isn't fat at all—it's **bloat and water retention.**

Let's be clear on the difference:

- **Fat gain** is gradual. It comes from a consistent caloric surplus over time.
- **Bloating and retention** are sudden. They shift throughout the day, often triggered by hormonal changes, dehydration, mineral imbalance, or poor digestion.

Pink salt helps you target these directly:

- **It balances sodium-potassium levels**, helping your body release excess water rather than hoard it.

- **It improves enzyme function and stomach acid**, reducing fermentation-based bloat after meals.
- **It lowers cortisol**, which is a major driver of belly puffiness—especially under stress.

When your belly softens and flattens mid-morning, not because of a workout, but because your body finally exhaled… That's not weight loss.
That's **inflammation loss.**
That's **stress relief.**
That's *hormonal harmony reclaiming space in your body.*

The Emotional Fatigue of Dieting—And How One Ritual Rebuilds Trust

There is a deep, invisible wound most women carry that few weight loss books talk about:

The trauma of being at war with your own body.

Years of tracking, punishing, restricting, and failing—not because you didn't try hard enough, but because the systems you followed were never designed with your biology in mind.

Every failed attempt chips away at your self-trust.
Every "start over Monday" feels heavier.
Every pound you gain back feels like personal failure.

The result? Emotional fatigue. Food shame. Decision paralysis.

The pink salt trick isn't a solution because it "works."
It's a healing ritual because it begins to rebuild something more sacred than weight loss: **self-trust.**

You wake up, and instead of running to fix your body, you nourish it.
You hydrate it.
You whisper to it, "I've *got you.*"

This one act of nourishment begins to unravel years of battle.

It's not a diet.
It's **a repair of the relationship** between you and the body that has carried you through everything.

The Psychology of "Morning Wins" & Momentum Stacking

Behavioral psychologists have proven something simple and profound:

> Tiny wins in the morning predict momentum for the rest of the day.

When you begin your day with a ritual that's easy, energizing, and embodied, it sets off a chain reaction:

- You make better breakfast choices
- You feel hydrated instead of foggy
- You crave less caffeine

- You move more
- You snack less at night

This is called **momentum stacking**—and it's exactly why the Pink Salt Ritual works beyond just biology. It gives you a consistent, early-day *win* that makes the rest of the day feel doable, even on the hardest mornings.

You don't need motivation.
You just need a **starting point that feels like self-care instead of self-control.**

That's the difference between forcing and flowing.
That's the difference between relapse and reset.

Breaking the Cycle—One Morning at a Time

If your days feel like a pendulum swinging between

- Fatigue and false energy
- Cravings and guilt
- Restriction and rebellion
- Swelling and shame

...it's time to break the cycle.

You don't have to overhaul everything.
You don't have to fix yourself.
You just have to begin—consistently, gently—with the ritual that

tells your body:
"We're not fighting anymore. We're listening now."

One glass.
One pinch.
One morning win.

And tomorrow, we'll show you how.

Because Chapter 4 is where the real magic begins—where we hand you the full, step-by-step Pink Salt Morning Ritual Blueprint. The timing, the upgrades, the customizations, the rhythm.

Not as another rule to follow.
But as a ritual to come home to.

Chapter 4

The 5-Minute Pink Salt Morning Ritual Blueprint

Let's simplify everything.

You don't need a 14-day detox.
You don't need a 10-supplement protocol.
You don't need a spreadsheet to fix your mornings.

What you need is a **ritual**—a rhythm so natural and effective that your body begins to *crave* it. Something you can do every single day, whether you're rushing out the door or enjoying a slow sunrise.

This is not just a drink. It's not just water and salt.
It's a metabolic message.
A hydration hug.
A nervous system nudge.
And a signal to your hormones: *We're starting today with nourishment, not deprivation.*

In this chapter, we break down every detail of the Pink Salt Morning Ritual—from the why behind each step to the optional upgrades that can transform it into a full-blown wellness practice in under five minutes.

Step-by-Step Pink Salt Morning Drink Routine

Here's the simplest version of the ritual that you can begin today:

You'll need:

- A glass of warm (not hot) filtered water (8 to 16 ounces)
- A pinch of high-quality Himalayan pink salt (about 1/8 teaspoon or less)

Instructions:

1. Fill your glass with warm filtered water.
2. Add a small pinch of pink Himalayan salt.
3. Stir until fully dissolved.
4. Sip slowly and mindfully—preferably within the first 30 minutes of waking, before coffee or food.

That's it.

This basic version delivers a potent, metabolic reset to your entire system. It begins the process of mineral replenishment, adrenal support, digestive priming, and hormonal balancing.

But like all powerful habits, this can evolve with you.

Best Times, Water Temperature, Salt Dosage & Upgrades

Best Timing

Drink your pink salt water within 5 to 30 minutes of waking. Why?

Because your body wakes up **dehydrated and depleted.** Overnight, you lose fluids through respiration, and your stress hormones (especially cortisol) are peaking in anticipation of the day.

This is your moment to intervene—**gently and strategically**—before the chaos of caffeine, phones, and meals begins.

Water Temperature

Use **warm or room-temperature** water. This supports digestion, relaxes the stomach, and increases absorption. Cold water can shock your system first thing and slow down the assimilation of minerals.

Warm water tells your body, "Wake *up gently." We're flowing today.*

Salt Dosage

Start small. You don't need a full teaspoon. Use just a **small pinch**—typically 1/8 teaspoon per 8 to 12 ounces of water.

If you feel bloated, sluggish, or especially depleted (e.g., post-workout, heavy sweating, traveling, low-carb eating), you can go up to 1/4 teaspoon. Always listen to your body. Less is often more when it comes to salt.

If you're concerned about taste, start with less and build up as your palate adjusts.

When & How to Customize Based on Energy or Goals

This ritual isn't one-size-fits-all. In fact, it works best when you tailor it to your needs and rhythms. Here are some ways to modify based on your current state:

Low Energy, Morning Brain Fog

Add a slice of fresh lemon and a few drops of liquid trace minerals or magnesium glycinate. This combination boosts alertness and supports cellular energy production.

Poor Sleep or Stress Hangover

Include a pinch of Celtic sea salt (alongside pink salt) and a few drops of calming herbs like ashwagandha tincture or tulsi tea infusion. This variation helps calm the adrenal system and soften cortisol peaks.

Constipation or Sluggish Digestion

Add a dash of apple cider vinegar (ACV) and a squeeze of ginger juice or ground ginger. These stimulate stomach acid and peristalsis—the muscle contractions that move your bowels.

Post-Workout or Sweat Recovery

Mix pink salt with coconut water or add potassium-rich ingredients like lemon or a banana on the side. This supports electrolyte replenishment and muscular repair.

These simple upgrades can transform your morning mineral water into a personalized wellness tonic.

Optional Add-Ons: Lemon, ACV, Trace Minerals, Ginger, etc.

The core ritual is powerful on its own—but these additions can offer extra support, flavor, and functional benefit:

- **Fresh Lemon Juice**—Adds vitamin C, alkalizes the body, and enhances taste. Also stimulates bile production and liver detox.
- **Apple Cider Vinegar (ACV)—Aids** digestion, balances blood sugar, and contains beneficial enzymes. Use just 1 tsp.
- **Trace Mineral Drops**—Support thyroid health, hydration, and metabolism.
- **Raw Honey**—For women with blood sugar crashes, a teaspoon of raw honey can calm adrenals and prevent dizziness.
- Ginger—Supports circulation and digestion and has anti-inflammatory properties.
- **Cayenne Pepper**—Boosts metabolism and circulation (use sparingly).
- Turmeric—Anti-inflammatory and powerful for liver support.

Keep your variations simple. Don't overwhelm the body. Treat your ritual like a sacred preparation, not a chemical cocktail.

Realistic Habit Stacking: How to Never Forget It Again

The key to sustainability is **integration**, not perfection.

This ritual becomes second nature when you attach it to existing anchors in your morning routine. Here's how to make it unskippable:

- **Put the salt and a clean glass beside your bed at night.** Prepare it before sleep so you wake up ready.
- **Make it your phone-unlock moment.** Don't check messages or social media until you've had your first sip.
- **Pair it with your journal, meditation, or sunlight exposure.** Let it become part of a calming, regulating rhythm.
- **Keep a pre-mixed bottle in the fridge or on your desk** for chaotic mornings.
- **Say a mantra or affirmation as you drink it.**
  "I am restoring. I am releasing. I am rising."

When a habit is built into your nervous system, it no longer requires motivation. It becomes identity.

The Ritual That Remembers You

This isn't a trend. It's a **return**—to the wisdom your body already knows. To the rhythm your ancestors honored. To the science that modern wellness is just now validating.

The Pink Salt Morning Ritual isn't just about metabolism or hydration.
It's about building **emotional momentum** in the first few moments of your day.

Before the emails.
Before the cravings.
Before the outside noise.

You begin with **presence**, **nourishment**, and **signaling safety** to your entire system.

That's not small.
That's everything.

And in the next chapter, we'll explore how this simple ritual does more than hydrate—it detoxifies without deprivation. We'll dive into liver function, lymphatic flow, and how pink salt gently resets the body without the crash-and-burn methods of most cleanse culture.

You don't need to purge.
You need to support.

And your minerals are ready to lead the way.

Chapter 5

Detox Without Deprivation—Salt, Liver & Lymph

Detox doesn't have to hurt.
You don't have to starve.
You don't need to buy a juice cleanse, swallow 20 supplements, or cancel your social life for 7 days.

Because real detoxification—the kind that makes your skin glow, your stomach flatten, and your energy hum—isn't about *removing more*. It's about *restoring what's missing.*

In this chapter, you'll discover how pink salt plays an overlooked but essential role in daily, sustainable detox. You'll learn why most cleanses fail, how mineral depletion backfires, and why your liver and lymphatic system respond better to nourishment than to punishment.

If you've ever done everything "right" and still felt heavy, puffy, foggy, or fatigued...
It's time to detox like your body actually wants you to.

How Pink Salt Supports Gentle Daily Detox

Let's reframe detox.

Your body is already designed to detox—every second of every day. Your **liver, kidneys, lymph, gut, skin, lungs, and even your tongue** are elimination organs. Their job? To neutralize, filter, and release what you no longer need.

But here's the problem:
Most women are trying to detox without the **raw materials** required to do it properly.

What's missing?

Minerals. Hydration. Flow. Support.

Pink salt supports detoxification in powerful yet gentle ways:

- **Replenishes essential electrolytes** required by detox enzymes in the liver
- **Hydrates cells more effectively**, allowing waste to exit more freely
- **Stimulates stomach acid and bile**, which aid in digesting and eliminating toxins
- **Supports adrenal function**, which prevents the stress-related slowdown of elimination

In other words, pink salt **doesn't force detox. It enables it.**

Think of it as giving your liver the keys to the car and a full tank of gas—not slamming the gas pedal with no oil in the engine.

Why Over-Cleansing Fails—And Mineral Depletion Backfires

We live in an era of aggressive detox marketing.

7-day juice fasts. 10-day master cleanses. Colon-blasting powders. Liquid-only diets.
And what do they all have in common?

They often leave you

- Dizzy
- Anxious
- Cold
- Constipated
- Binge-prone
- And back where you started

Here's why: most "cleanses" are missing minerals.

When you flush your body without replenishing sodium, potassium, magnesium, and chloride, you disrupt fluid balance, slow your metabolism, and **stress your detox organs.** The liver in particular depends on minerals to function properly:

- **Magnesium** is required for over 300 detox pathways.
- **Sodium** powers the sodium-potassium pump that moves waste out of cells.

- **Zinc and selenium** help with phase 2 liver detoxification.
- **Chloride**, naturally present in pink salt, helps maintain pH balance in the blood and supports digestion.

So while green juices and teas might make you feel virtuous, without minerals, you're just *leaking out energy*, not releasing waste.

That's why the Pink Salt Ritual works. It **supports your body's daily detox work**—without draining your reserves.

The Lymphatic System, Salt Baths & Morning Movement

The liver is your chemical detox organ.
But your lymphatic system? That's your **physical drainage network.**

The lymph system is a vast web of vessels and nodes that flush out cellular waste, dead bacteria, metabolic byproducts, and inflammatory compounds. But unlike your heart, your lymph doesn't pump on its own. It needs movement and hydration to flow.

That's where pink salt comes in.

Mineral Hydration for Lymph Flow

Lymph fluid is 95% water—but it also depends on **osmotic pressure** and **electrolyte balance** to move. Dehydration or mineral imbalance causes lymph stagnation, which shows up as:

- Puffy eyes

- Swollen ankles
- Cellulite
- Tender underarms or neck
- Fatigue and fogginess

Pink salt provides the electrolytes your body needs to keep lymph flowing efficiently, especially first thing in the morning.

Salt Baths as Lymph Detox Therapy

Soaking in a hot bath with pink Himalayan salt can stimulate lymph movement and skin detoxification through:

- **Reverse osmosis**: Drawing toxins out of the skin
- **Muscle relaxation**: Allowing smoother fluid flow
- **Improved circulation**: Especially when combined with essential oils or gentle scrubbing

Just one 20-minute bath with 1–2 cups of pink salt can feel like an internal shower—leaving you lighter, calmer, and clearer.

Morning Movement: Walking, Rebounding, or Dry Brushing

Your lymph doesn't need high-intensity cardio. It needs **gentle rhythm.** The best time to activate lymphatic drainage is right after your morning salt drink.

Simple ways to activate lymph flow:

- **5–10 minutes of light stretching** or yoga
- **Rebounding** on a mini-trampoline (2–5 minutes)
- **Dry brushing** toward the heart before a shower
- **Brisk morning walk in fresh air**

When pink salt, hydration, and movement combine, you create a **daily detox trifecta**—no powders, starvation, or pain required.

Hydration Myths That Hurt Weight Loss

You've probably heard the advice: *"Drink more water."*

But the truth is, **plain water alone can dehydrate you.**

That sounds counterintuitive, but here's the science: when you drink large amounts of water without replenishing **electrolytes**, especially sodium, your body:

- Dilutes your blood sodium levels (hyponatremia)
- Increases urination without increasing true hydration
- Puts pressure on the kidneys and adrenal system
- Signals the body to hold onto water—causing *bloating*, not flushing

That's why some women feel more bloated and tired the more water they drink. It's not the water—it's the **lack of minerals** in the water.

Pink salt turns your water into a **hydration solution** that your cells can absorb and use. It's like upgrading from a dusty hose to a pressurized irrigation system.

The result?

- Better bowel movements
- Flatter stomach
- Improved skin tone
- Fewer headaches
- Less puffiness

So if you're drinking water all day but still feel sluggish or swollen, it's time to **salt smarter.**

24-Hour Salt-Supported Body Reset Protocol

Ready for a gentle, full-day metabolic reset using the principles of this chapter?

Here's a realistic flow you can follow anytime you feel heavy, inflamed, or off-track—no starvation, no supplements, no guilt:

Morning

- **Wake**: Pink Salt Morning Ritual (warm water + pinch of Himalayan salt + lemon or trace minerals)
- **Move:** 10-minute walk or stretch while breathing deeply
- **Cleanse:** Dry brush before your shower

- Eat a light, protein-rich breakfast with anti-inflammatory fats (eggs + avocado or hemp seeds + smoothie)

Midday

- **Hydrate:** Refill your bottle with mineral water (add another pinch of salt if needed)
- Eat a nourishing, mineral-rich meal (like broth-based soup, greens, and salmon or lentils)
- **Optional:** Sip detox tea (dandelion, ginger, nettle) between meals

Evening

- **Relax:** Take a warm bath with 1–2 cups pink salt and a few drops of lavender or eucalyptus oil
- Eat a light, cooked dinner—focus on fiber and digestion (roasted veggies + brown rice + herbs)
- **Sip:** Bedtime salt tonic (warm water + trace pink salt + honey + turmeric for calm)

This gentle reset supports elimination, reduces inflammation, and restores clarity—all without stress, hunger, or deprivation.

Do it once a week or after stressful periods. It's a return, not a punishment.

Detox Isn't a Fight—It's a Flow

You are not a toxic swamp.
You are a self-healing, self-cleansing organism—one that needs **support**, not war.

The pink salt trick works because it doesn't force. It **frees**.

It reminds your liver it has what it needs.
It nudges your lymph to move.
It turns water into medicine.
It teaches your body to trust again.

And now that your foundation is nourished, your metabolism reset, your cravings softened, and your system flowing…

It's time to eat.

Chapter 6

The Pink Salt Diet—Simple, Nourishing Meals That Work

What if the best "diet" isn't a diet at all?

No calorie counting.
No macro math.
No guilt-tripping checklists.
No food rules wrapped in wellness disguise.

Just meals that feel nourishing. Satisfying. Calm.
Just food that supports your body's chemistry, not manipulates it.

This chapter isn't about restricting your plate. It's about *rewiring* the relationship between salt, satisfaction, digestion, and true nourishment. You'll learn how pink salt becomes a tool of metabolic awareness—not a flavor bomb or a trend. You'll discover the simple foods that work in synergy with salt to curb cravings, reduce bloat, and support fat loss—without a shred of restriction.

This is **not** a diet. It's a **return to intuitive nourishment**... anchored in mineral wisdom.

The Diet That Isn't a Diet: Salt as the Foundation

The word "diet" has become synonymous with deprivation, discipline, and disconnection. But its root meaning, from the Greek *diaita*, simply means **"way of life."**

The Pink Salt Diet isn't about following rules. It's about **building meals around what your body truly needs: minerals, balance, and calm.**

Pink salt becomes the starting point, not the center of every dish. Its role is to:

- **Stimulate digestion** so your body actually absorbs nutrients
- **Regulate hydration and fullness**, reducing cravings and bloating
- **Enhance flavor** so meals feel satisfying and complete without overeating.
- **Signal satiety** through neural and hormonal feedback

When you begin with a pinch of pink salt—whether in water, on roasted vegetables, or in broth—you're sending a signal:
"We're about to eat. Digest. Absorb. Heal."

That single shift changes the tone of your entire day.

Anti-Inflammatory Foods That Synergize with Pink Salt

To maximize the benefits of pink salt for weight loss and hormonal balance, pair it with foods that **lower inflammation**, stabilize blood sugar, and support the gut.

Here are the foods that *love* pink salt—and help you thrive:

Leafy Greens & Sulfur-Rich Veggies

Spinach, kale, arugula, broccoli, cabbage, cauliflower
Rich in chlorophyll, fiber, and compounds that support liver detox and estrogen metabolism. Pink salt enhances their flavor while helping you absorb their minerals.

Healthy Fats

Avocados, extra virgin olive oil, wild-caught salmon, hemp seeds, walnuts
These fats slow glucose absorption, calm the nervous system, and help shuttle fat-soluble nutrients. Salt deepens the satisfaction factor, reducing the urge to snack later.

Clean Proteins

Organic eggs, grass-fed beef, lentils, tempeh, turkey, sardines
Protein builds lean muscle and balances blood sugar. Salt activates taste buds and digestive enzymes, helping you absorb amino acids more efficiently.

Root Vegetables & Slow Carbs

Sweet potatoes, carrots, beets, quinoa, wild rice
Complex carbs are not the enemy—they're fuel for thyroid and hormone balance. When salted properly and cooked with healthy fats, they leave you grounded, not groggy.

Ferments & Digestive Boosters

Kimchi, sauerkraut, lemon, apple cider vinegar, ginger
These support digestion, reduce bloating, and restore gut flora. A pinch of salt in lemon water or ACV boosts their effects.

When you combine these foods with pink salt in intuitive, satisfying meals, you stop fighting your food.
You begin *partnering* with it.

How to Eat Without Fear, Counting, or Restriction

Let's be clear: you don't need another set of "good vs. bad" food rules. You've had enough of those.

Instead, adopt these five soul-nourishing principles:

1. Salt Before Sugar

Start your day and your meals with minerals, not glucose. This means pink salt water in the morning and protein + fat + veggies before carbs or fruit. Doing this blunts the insulin spike and reduces post-meal crashes.

2. Cooked Over Cold

Warm, cooked meals with salt are easier to digest and assimilate. Cold raw salads may sound virtuous but often lead to bloating. Salted stews, soups, and roasted veggies are grounding and nourishing.

3. Eat When You're Hungry, Not Empty

True hunger is grounded and grows slowly. Emotional eating is frantic and urgent. Pink salt helps you tune in. Craving a second helping? Pause. Sip salt water. Breathe. Reconnect.

4. Flavor = Satisfaction

Don't fear seasoning. Salt, herbs, garlic, and lemon—these are tools of deep satisfaction. When food tastes good and feels good, you naturally eat enough—not too much.

5. Trust Takes Time

You won't instantly wake up one day with a perfect intuitive eating voice. But every salted morning, every satisfying lunch, every calm evening snack—you rebuild trust. One bite at a time.

Pink Salt Timing with Meals (and When Not to Use It)

Timing matters—not for calories, but for chemistry. Here's how to time pink salt throughout the day to maximize its benefits:

Morning

Drink pink salt water 15–30 minutes before eating. This primes digestion, supports adrenal function, and sets the tone for balanced energy.

With Meals

Sprinkle a modest amount of pink salt on your food—not as an afterthought, but as a **pre-digestive signal.** Salt stimulates salivary enzymes and stomach acid production.

Deal with:

- Cooked vegetables
- Bone broths
- Steamed grains
- Light Proteins: When **Not to Use**

Avoid heavy salt use late at night, especially if you're prone to water retention or insomnia. Salt can slightly elevate aldosterone and cortisol if taken too close to sleep. Instead, opt for calming blends (like pink salt with magnesium and warm herbal tea).

Also avoid excessive pink salt with:

- Ultra-processed foods (which already contain sodium)
- High-sodium snacks like deli meats or canned soups
- Salt "pill" supplements unless medically advised

Use pink salt as a **ritual**, not a reaction.

Understanding True Hunger vs. Salt-Triggered Satisfaction

You've been taught to associate fullness with fullness of stomach. But true satisfaction is **neurological**—it's about what signals your brain receives after a meal.

Salt plays a fascinating role here:

- **Enhances leptin signaling**, helping your brain register satiety
- **Improves insulin sensitivity**, which lowers post-meal cravings
- **Calms cortisol**, which reduces stress-eating tendencies
- **Activates taste receptors**, which satisfy the sensory experience of eating

In short, food tastes better, satisfies faster, and sits more calmly in your body when it's seasoned with intention.

To test this:
Next time you eat, try a bite with salt. Then one without.
Notice how quickly the unsalted bite becomes boring or unsatisfying.

Salt isn't just flavor—it's a **neural cue that says, "We're complete."**

A Sample Pink Salt Day of Eating (No Counting, No Chaos)

Morning

- Pink salt lemon water
- Scrambled eggs cooked in olive oil with spinach and sea salt
- Half avocado with crushed hemp seeds and a pinch of pink salt

Midday

- Slow-cooked lentil and root vegetable stew with pink salt, turmeric, garlic, and rosemary
- Side of fermented carrots or sauerkraut
- Warm mineral tea with lemon and ginger

Afternoon Snack

- Apple slices with tahini and a dash of pink salt
- Or a soft-boiled egg and cucumber slices with a sprinkle of paprika and salt

Evening

- Baked wild salmon or chickpea patties
- Roasted zucchini, squash, and red onion with olive oil and pink salt

- Small portion of brown rice with ghee and parsley
- Herbal bedtime drink with pink salt, turmeric, and honey

Reclaiming the Joy of Eating

You've been told that food is the problem.
But the real problem is the fear that's been built around food.

The Pink Salt Diet isn't a prescription. It's a **permission**—to return to the kind of eating your body remembers. Meals with minerals. Flavor. Calm. Warmth. Wholeness.

No apps. No labels. No punishment.

That trust is being rebuilt, meal by mineral-rich meal.
And now that you're nourished from the inside out, it's time to put everything together into a transformative 3-week rhythm.

Because next up: **The 21-Day Pink Salt Metabolic Reset Plan**—a full daily ritual blueprint that takes everything you've learned so far and turns it into sustainable results.

You're ready.

Chapter 7

The 21-Day Pink Salt Metabolic Reset Plan

This isn't another plan to follow.

This is the beginning of a rhythm that remembers who you were before the diets, before the scale, before the fatigue.

You're not here to track your way thin.
You're here to return to balance.

The **21-Day Pink Salt Metabolic Reset** isn't about perfection. It's about **retraining your body to trust again**—with consistent nourishment, mineral-rich rituals, and micro-habits that create sustainable fat loss, better energy, and hormonal healing.

This chapter will give you everything you need to shift from survival mode to metabolic resilience in 3 gentle, powerful phases: **Cleanse, Balance, and Thrive.**

No obsession. No starvation. No restriction.

Just a daily rhythm that feels real—and works.

Why 21 Days?

Why not 7? Or 30?

Because **21 days** is long enough to:

- Reprogram your stress response
- Improve digestion, hydration, and sleep
- Reset your relationship with cravings
- Trigger visible changes in energy, bloating, and weight

But it's also short enough to feel doable—and flexible. You're not committing to forever. You're creating **a reset window**—one where you finally feel safe enough to stop forcing your body and start listening to it.

This plan isn't rigid. It's intelligent. And it's built around **consistency, not control.**

Overview of the 3 Phases

PHASE 1: CLEANSE (Days 1–7)

Goal: Reduce inflammation, reset digestion, and begin morning mineral rituals.

PHASE 2: BALANCE (Days 8–14)

Goal: Rebuild metabolic trust, reduce cravings, and normalize hunger cues.

PHASE 3: THRIVE (Days 15–21)

Goal: Improve energy output, deepen body awareness, and sustain results without rules.

Each phase builds on the last. Let's break them down.

PHASE 1: CLEANSE (DAYS 1–7)

Focus: Simplify. Reset. Reduce internal noise.

This week is about **removing metabolic interference**—bloating, overstimulation, blood sugar crashes, dehydration, and chaotic eating rhythms.

Daily Musts:

- **Pink Salt Morning Ritual**: Every day upon waking (warm water + pink salt + optional lemon or trace minerals)
- **Anti-inflammatory meals**: simple proteins, cooked veggies, and healthy fats. No processed sugar or alcohol.
- **30 mins light movement**: Walking, stretching, yoga—just enough to stimulate lymph flow and digestion
- **Hydration reset**: Minimum 2 liters per day of mineral-rich water
- **Salt bath or foot soak** 2–3 times this week to aid lymphatic drainage

Optional Enhancements:

- Herbal teas (nettle, dandelion, ginger)
- Journaling: *How does my body feel today—before and after salt?*

PHASE 2: BALANCE (DAYS 8–14)

Focus: Rebuild metabolic harmony.

This is where things begin to shift. Cravings lessen. Sleep deepens. Your belly feels lighter. This week is about **stabilizing blood sugar, reactivating natural hunger cues**, and building satiety.

Daily Musts:

- Continue **Morning Pink Salt Ritual**
- Start meals with **protein, fat, and fiber** before carbs
- **Include sea vegetables or magnesium-rich greens** once per day
- **Hydration** with intentional salt dosage based on sweat, cycle, or energy
- 10-minute **morning walk** to re-sync circadian rhythm

Optional Upgrades:

- Salt-enhanced broth midday to support adrenal resilience

- Bitters or lemon water before meals to stimulate bile flow

PHASE 3: THRIVE (DAYS 15–21)

Focus: Strengthen metabolism and maintain without force.

Now the body is recalibrated. You've reduced bloat, softened cravings, and deepened energy. It's time to add back variety and **build sustainability into your flow.**

Daily Musts:

- Continue **Morning Ritual**
- **Expand your meals**—more flavors, more colors, more joy
- Add **gentle resistance training** 2–3x (bodyweight, bands, light weights)
- Stay **salt-conscious**, but don't obsess—your body is now better at signaling
- Begin **habit layering**: pairing salt with gratitude, movement, silence

Optional Expansions:

- Try a new recipe from Chapter 8
- Walk in sunlight before or after a mineralized meal
- Reflect on emotional patterns you've released

Weekly Goals, Mindset Prompts & Measurable Wins

Each phase has specific **outcomes** to celebrate:

Phase	Physical Wins	Emotional Wins
Cleanse	Flatter stomach, fewer crashes, better sleep	Clarity, calm, breaking food obsession
Balance	Reduced cravings, regular digestion	Trust in hunger/fullness, reduced stress
Thrive	Visible energy shifts, better skin	Joyful eating, sustainable routines

You can measure your wins in how your clothes fit, how steady your energy feels, and how little food fear you experience—not in numbers.

Daily Rituals, Meal Ideas & Micro-Challenges

You don't need a meal plan. You need meal patterns. Here's a rhythm to follow and adapt:

Mornings:

- Pink salt water
- Protein- and fat-rich breakfast (e.g., eggs + avocado or hemp protein + almond butter smoothie)
- 5–10 minutes of light movement or sunlight exposure

Midday:

- Hydrating broth or tea
- Warm, mineral-rich meal with clean protein, greens, fat, and slow carbs
- Digestive pause: walk, stretch, breathe

Evenings:

- Calming dinner with cooked vegetables and mineral seasoning
- No screens while eating
- Optional: warm pink salt & honey bedtime drink

Micro-challenges to layer in:

- Go one day completely screen-free during meals
- Prepare one meal mindfully from scratch
- Walk after every meal for 5 minutes
- Share your ritual with someone else

This is how rituals become identity. This is how healing becomes a lifestyle.

How to Adjust If You're Not Losing Weight (Troubleshooting)

Plateau? Here's what to check before you panic:

Are you...

- Drinking enough **mineralized water**?
- Eating **enough food**? (Undereating slows metabolism.)
- Sleeping at least 7 hours?

- Managing **stress** or spiking cortisol daily?
- Getting **gentle movement** in the mornings?

Reset tweaks:

- Add 1 more cup of warm water with pink salt mid-afternoon
- Eliminate sugar "sneaks" (flavored yogurts, bars, etc.)
- Add bitters or ACV 15 minutes before meals
- Do a salt bath nightly for 3 days to clear stagnation

Remember, weight is one marker. Fat loss, inflammation release, energy, and digestion matter more.

Maintaining Results Without "Staying on a Plan"

You're not here to be on a plan forever. You're here to live light.

When the 21 days are complete, ask:

- What rituals feel natural to keep?
- What foods leave me feeling calm and steady?
- Where did I feel the most emotional relief?

Keep those. Let go of the rest.

The Pink Salt Reset is not a trap—it's a bridge. A way back to your body's knowing. And from this place, you get to **live**, not just follow.

Next, in Chapter 8, you'll unlock **101 Pink Salt Recipes**—not as rules, but as inspiration. Recipes that help you burn fat, calm cravings, boost digestion, and glow from within—all mineralized, nourishing, and full of joy.

Because now? You're not starting over.
You're building a life that begins with salt—and ends in balance.

Chapter 8

101 Pink Salt Recipes for Weight Loss & Wellness

You don't need another diet plan.
You need meals and drinks that *love you back.*

That calms your gut.
That energizes without crashing.
That tastes good, feels grounding, and leaves you lighter—not just physically, but emotionally.

This chapter is your pink salt kitchen—a collection of **101 practical, nourishing, metabolism-supporting recipes** to make your reset delicious and deeply sustainable. You'll find simple, fat-burning morning drinks, gut-soothing smoothies, debloating soups, satisfying mineral-rich meals, and calming bedtime tonics—each infused with the grounding wisdom of **Himalayan pink salt.**

Whether you need a fast craving fix or a gentle hormone-supportive broth, it's all here.

No calorie counts.
No tracking.
Just rituals in recipe form.

A. Fat-Burning Pink Salt Morning Drinks

These drinks jumpstart hydration, fat-burning, and mineral balance. Drink them first thing in the morning, ideally before food or caffeine.

1. Classic Pink Salt & Lemon Elixir

Ingredients:

- 1 glass of warm filtered water
- 1/8 teaspoon pink Himalayan salt
- Juice of ½ lemon

How to Make:
Fill your glass with warm water. Stir in the pink salt until it fully dissolves. Squeeze in fresh lemon juice. Stir again. Drink slowly on an empty stomach.

2. Pink Salt Warm Ginger Water

Ingredients:

- 1 cup warm water
- 1/8 teaspoon pink salt
- 3 slices of fresh ginger or 1/4 teaspoon grated ginger

How to Make:
Bring water to a gentle simmer. Add ginger and let steep for 5–7 minutes. Stir in pink salt. Drink warm.

3. Pink Salt & Apple Cider Vinegar Morning Tonic

Ingredients:

- 1 cup warm water
- 1 tablespoon raw, unfiltered apple cider vinegar
- 1/8 teaspoon pink salt

How to Make:
Stir pink salt and apple cider vinegar into warm water until fully mixed. Drink slowly, 15–30 minutes before breakfast.

4. Pink Salt Electrolyte Lemonade

Ingredients:

- 1 tall glass of cold or room-temperature water
- Juice of 1 lemon
- 1/8 teaspoon pink salt
- Optional: a few drops of liquid stevia or raw honey

How to Make:
Stir all ingredients together in a glass or shake in a sealed jar. Drink it chilled or at room temperature for a refreshing wake-up.

5. Lemon-Ginger Pink Salt Hydration Shot

Ingredients:

- ½ cup warm water
- ½ teaspoon grated ginger
- Juice of ½ lemon
- 1 pinch pink salt

How to Make:
Combine all ingredients in a small glass. Stir well. Drink it like a wellness shot.

6. Cucumber Mint Morning Flush

Ingredients:

- 1 glass room temperature water
- 2 cucumber slices
- 3 mint leaves
- 1/8 teaspoon pink salt
- Juice of ½ lime or lemon

How to Make:
Crush mint leaves slightly to release aroma. Add everything into the water and stir. Let it sit for 2 minutes before drinking.

7. Pink Salt Honey-Cayenne Booster

Ingredients:

- 1 cup warm water

- 1/8 teaspoon pink salt
- 1 teaspoon raw honey
- A small pinch of cayenne pepper

How to Make:
Stir pink salt and honey into warm water until dissolved. Add cayenne, stir again, and drink warm.

8. Salted Coconut Water with Lime

Ingredients:

- 1 cup unsweetened coconut water
- Juice of ½ lime
- Pinch of pink salt

How to Make:
Mix everything in a glass. Stir well. Drink cold or at room temp. Great post-workout or first thing in the morning.

9. Orange & Pink Salt Sunshine Juice

Ingredients:

- Juice of 1 fresh orange
- ½ cup water
- 1/8 teaspoon pink salt

How to Make:
Squeeze fresh orange into a glass. Add water and salt. Stir gently. Drink slowly to absorb the vitamin C and minerals.

10. Cinnamon Pink Salt Fat Burn Tonic

Ingredients:

- 1 cup warm water
- ½ teaspoon ground cinnamon
- 1/8 teaspoon pink salt
- Optional: 1 teaspoon apple cider vinegar

How to Make:
Mix cinnamon and salt into warm water. Stir thoroughly. Add ACV if desired. Sip it warm in the morning.

11. Morning Magnesium Tea with Pink Salt

Ingredients:

- 1 cup herbal tea (e.g., rooibos, chamomile, or mint))
- 1/8 teaspoon pink salt
- Optional: magnesium glycinate powder (check dosage)

How to Make:
Brew your herbal tea. Stir in salt and optional magnesium powder. Drink slowly in the morning to calm adrenals.

12. Salted Warm Turmeric Lemon Water

Ingredients:

- 1 cup warm water
- ½ teaspoon turmeric powder
- Juice of ½ lemon
- Pinch of pink salt
- Pinch of black pepper

How to Make:
Mix all ingredients in a mug. Stir well and drink warm. This helps inflammation and digestion.

13. Pink Salt Chia Detox Hydrator

Ingredients:

- 1 glass water
- 1 tablespoon chia seeds
- Juice of ½ lemon
- 1/8 teaspoon pink salt

How to Make:
Add chia to water and let it sit for 10–15 minutes to form a gel. Add salt and lemon juice. Stir and drink.

14. Pink Salt + Chlorophyll Morning Cleanser

Ingredients:

- 1 cup water
- 1 dropper chlorophyll liquid
- 1/8 teaspoon pink salt

How to Make:
Stir chlorophyll and salt into water. Drink chilled or at room temperature. Ideal for cellular detox.

15. Aloe Vera & Pink Salt Digestion Tonic

Ingredients:

- ½ cup aloe vera juice (unsweetened, inner leaf only)
- ½ cup water
- Juice of ½ lemon
- Pinch of pink salt

How to Make:
Mix all ingredients in a glass. Stir thoroughly. Drink before meals or first thing in the morning.

B. Gut-Friendly Detox Smoothies with Salt Integration

16. Avocado Lime Salted Smoothie

Ingredients:

- ½ ripe avocado
- Juice of ½ lime
- 1 handful baby spinach
- 1 cup coconut water or almond milk
- 1/8 teaspoon pink salt
- Optional: ice cubes

How to Make:
Add all ingredients into a blender. Blend until smooth and creamy. Add ice if desired. Drink immediately for a creamy, satisfying, gut-loving smoothie.

17. Salted Pineapple Ginger Gut Cleanse

Ingredients:

- 1 cup fresh pineapple chunks
- ½ inch piece of fresh ginger (peeled)
- ½ banana

- 1 cup water or coconut water
- 1/8 teaspoon pink salt

How to Make:
Blend all ingredients until smooth. Drink cold. The enzymes in pineapple combined with ginger and salt help reduce inflammation and support digestion.

18. Pink Salt & Green Apple Fiber Flush

Ingredients:

- 1 green apple, cored
- 1 handful kale or spinach
- Juice of ½ lemon
- 1 tablespoon chia seeds
- 1 cup water
- Pinch of pink salt

How to Make:
Blend apple, greens, lemon juice, chia seeds, water, and salt until fully smooth. Let it sit for 2 minutes to thicken slightly before drinking.

19. Banana Almond Mineral Shake

Ingredients:

- 1 banana (fresh or frozen)
- 1 tablespoon almond butter
- 1 cup unsweetened almond milk
- 1/8 teaspoon pink salt
- Dash of cinnamon (optional)

How to Make:
Blend everything together until smooth. Enjoy chilled. This creamy blend is excellent for hormone support and blood sugar balance.

20. Papaya Mint Debloat Smoothie

Ingredients:

- 1 cup ripe papaya cubes
- ½ cucumber
- 3 mint leaves
- 1/2 cup coconut water
- 1/8 teaspoon pink salt
- Juice of ½ lime

How to Make:
Blend until smooth. Drink cold. Papaya enzymes and mint soothe the digestive tract, while pink salt restores mineral balance.

21. Berry Beet Salted Smoothie

Ingredients:

- 1 small cooked beet (peeled)
- ½ cup mixed frozen berries
- 1 cup water or almond milk
- 1/8 teaspoon pink salt
- Optional: ½ banana for sweetness

How to Make:
Add everything into a blender and blend until vibrant and smooth. This antioxidant-rich smoothie supports liver and lymphatic flow.

22. Cucumber Parsley Liver Support Blend

Ingredients:

- ½ cucumber
- 1 tablespoon fresh parsley
- Juice of ½ lemon
- 1 cup water
- Pinch of pink salt
- Optional: 1 teaspoon honey

How to Make:
Blend all ingredients until fully liquefied. Drink chilled. This is a refreshing way to gently support liver function and reduce puffiness.

23. Salted Spinach & Pineapple Green Smoothie

Ingredients:

- 1 cup spinach
- ½ cup pineapple
- ½ frozen banana
- 1 cup water
- 1/8 teaspoon pink salt

How to Make:
Blend until smooth. This tropical-flavored smoothie hydrates while delivering key minerals and natural enzymes.

24. Watermelon Basil Mineral Smoothie

Ingredients:

- 1 cup fresh watermelon cubes
- 2 fresh basil leaves
- ½ cup coconut water
- Juice of ½ lime

- 1/8 teaspoon pink salt

How to Make:
Blend until liquefied. Drink immediately for hydration, mineral support, and a touch of summer.

25. Celery Pear Pink Salt Blend

Ingredients:

- 1 pear, chopped
- 1 stalk celery
- ½ inch ginger (peeled)
- 1 cup water
- Pinch of pink salt

How to Make:
Blend until smooth. This slightly sweet, slightly savory blend reduces bloating and boosts gut motility.

26. Blueberry Chia Balance Shake

Ingredients:

- ½ cup frozen blueberries
- 1 tablespoon chia seeds
- 1 cup almond milk or water
- 1/8 teaspoon pink salt

- Optional: 1 teaspoon raw honey

How to Make:
Blend all ingredients thoroughly. Let it sit for 3 minutes to thicken slightly, then enjoy. A powerful combo for blood sugar stability and fullness.

27. Creamy Cashew & Pink Salt Breakfast Shake

Ingredients:

- 1 tablespoon soaked cashews (or cashew butter)
- 1 small frozen banana
- 1 cup almond or oat milk
- 1/8 teaspoon pink salt
- Dash of vanilla extract (optional)

How to Make:
Blend until creamy. This satisfying shake keeps you full and supports adrenal function in the early morning.

28. Zucchini Banana Morning Blend

Ingredients:

- ½ raw zucchini (peeled)
- ½ banana
- 1 tablespoon flaxseed

- 1 cup almond milk
- 1/8 teaspoon pink salt

How to Make:
Blend until smooth. A surprisingly delicious way to sneak in greens and fiber.

29. Coconut Pink Salt Electrolyte Smoothie

Ingredients:

- ½ cup coconut milk
- ½ cup coconut water
- 1 frozen banana
- 1/8 teaspoon pink salt
- Optional: a pinch of cinnamon

How to Make:
Blend everything until frothy. Excellent for post-workout recovery or rehydration on detox days.

30. Salted Turmeric Mango Immune Smoothie

Ingredients:

- ½ cup frozen mango
- ½ teaspoon turmeric
- 1 cup almond milk

- 1/8 teaspoon pink salt
- Dash of black pepper (to activate turmeric)

How to Make:
Blend until vibrant yellow and smooth. A healing, anti-inflammatory powerhouse.

C. Pink Salt Soups, Stews & Savory Cravings Cures

31. Pink Salt Butternut Ginger Soup

Ingredients:

- 1 small butternut squash (peeled, cubed)
- 1 tablespoon olive oil
- 1 teaspoon grated fresh ginger
- 3 cups vegetable broth
- 1/2 teaspoon pink salt
- Optional: pinch of nutmeg or cinnamon

How to Make:
Sauté ginger in olive oil for 1–2 minutes. Add squash and stir. Pour in broth and bring to a boil. Reduce heat and simmer until squash is tender (about 20 minutes). Blend until smooth. Stir in pink salt. Serve warm.

32. Broccoli Leek Detox Soup

Ingredients:

- 1 leek (cleaned, sliced)
- 1 head of broccoli (chopped)
- 1 garlic clove (minced)
- 1 tablespoon olive oil
- 3 cups water or veggie broth
- 1/2 teaspoon pink salt

How to Make:
Sauté leek and garlic in olive oil. Add broccoli and liquid. Simmer for 15 minutes. Blend until silky. Add pink salt to taste.

33. Gut-Healing Carrot Turmeric Puree

Ingredients:

- 4 carrots (peeled, chopped)
- 1 teaspoon turmeric
- 1/8 teaspoon black pepper
- 2 cups vegetable broth
- 1/2 teaspoon pink salt

How to Make:
Simmer carrots, turmeric, pepper, and broth until carrots are soft. Blend until smooth. Stir in pink salt before serving.

34. Cabbage & Pink Salt Metabolism Stew

Ingredients:

- 1/2 head green cabbage (sliced)
- 1 carrot (sliced)
- 1 tomato (diced)
- 2 garlic cloves
- 3 cups broth or water
- 1/2 teaspoon pink salt
- 1 teaspoon apple cider vinegar

How to Make:
Add everything to a pot. Simmer for 25 minutes until soft. Adjust salt and vinegar to taste. This stew helps reduce bloating and supports liver health.

35. Coconut Cauliflower Curry with Salted Herbs

Ingredients:

- 1/2 head cauliflower (cut into florets)
- 1/2 cup coconut milk

- 1 teaspoon curry powder
- 1/2 teaspoon pink salt
- 1 cup water
- Chopped cilantro for garnish

How to Make:
Simmer cauliflower in water and coconut milk. Add curry powder and pink salt. Cook until tender. Serve topped with herbs.

36. Lentil & Sweet Potato Pink Salt Bowl

Ingredients:

- 1/2 cup lentils (rinsed)
- 1 small sweet potato (cubed)
- 3 cups water or broth
- 1/2 teaspoon pink salt
- Spices: cumin, turmeric, black pepper

How to Make:
Simmer lentils, sweet potato, and spices in water for 25–30 minutes. Stir in pink salt. This hearty bowl is full of fiber and grounding energy.

37. Spicy Salted Miso Veggie Soup

Ingredients:

- 1 tablespoon miso paste
- 1 cup chopped mushrooms
- 1 cup shredded greens (bok choy or kale)
- 2 cups water
- Pinch of pink salt
- Dash of chili flakes (optional)

How to Make:
Bring water to a simmer. Add veggies. Cook 5–7 minutes. Turn off the heat and stir in miso paste and pink salt. Do not boil miso. Serve hot.

38. Chickpea Tomato Pink Salt Stew

Ingredients:

- 1 cup canned or cooked chickpeas
- 1 tomato (chopped)
- 1 garlic clove
- 1/2 teaspoon paprika
- 1/2 teaspoon pink salt
- 1.5 cups water or broth

How to Make:
Sauté garlic and tomato in olive oil. Add chickpeas and broth. Simmer for 15 minutes. Stir in paprika and salt before serving.

39. Green Detox Soup with Spinach & Celery

Ingredients:

- 1 cup spinach
- 2 stalks celery
- 1 zucchini (chopped)
- 1 clove garlic
- 2 cups water
- 1/2 teaspoon pink salt

How to Make:
Boil all veggies until soft (about 10–15 minutes). Blend until smooth. Add pink salt to taste. Serve warm.

40. Roasted Garlic & Pink Salt Bone Broth

Ingredients:

- 3 cups bone broth
- 1 head roasted garlic (squeezed out)
- 1/2 teaspoon pink salt
- Optional: herbs like rosemary or thyme

How to Make:
Heat broth and stir in roasted garlic. Add pink salt. Let it simmer gently for 5 minutes. Sip it like a mineral-rich tea.

41. Zucchini Basil Puree with Lemon Salt

Ingredients:

- 2 zucchinis (chopped)
- 1 handful fresh basil
- Juice of 1/2 lemon
- 2 cups water
- 1/2 teaspoon pink salt

How to Make:
Boil zucchini until soft. Blend with basil and lemon juice. Stir in salt before serving. A light, fresh soup.

42. Cleansing Mushroom Seaweed Broth

Ingredients:

- 1 cup sliced mushrooms
- 1 teaspoon dried seaweed (wakame or dulse)
- 2 cups water
- 1/2 teaspoon pink salt
- Optional: sliced scallion

How to Make:
Simmer mushrooms and seaweed for 10 minutes. Add pink salt. Top with scallions before serving.

43. Pink Salt Sautéed Bok Choy with Ginger

Ingredients:

- 1 bunch bok choy (sliced)
- 1 teaspoon fresh ginger (grated)
- 1 teaspoon olive oil
- 1/4 teaspoon pink salt

How to Make:
Sauté ginger in oil. Add bok choy and stir-fry for 3–4 minutes until wilted. Sprinkle pink salt before serving.

44. Warming Pink Salt Turmeric Chickpea Soup

Ingredients:

- 1 cup cooked chickpeas
- 1/2 teaspoon turmeric
- 2 cups water or broth
- 1/2 teaspoon pink salt
- Pinch of black pepper

How to Make:
Simmer chickpeas with turmeric and broth for 15 minutes. Add salt and pepper before serving.

45. Carrot-Coriander Pink Salt Soup

Ingredients:

- 3 carrots (chopped)
- 1 teaspoon ground coriander
- 1 garlic clove
- 2 cups broth
- 1/2 teaspoon pink salt

How to Make:
Simmer carrots and garlic until soft. Add coriander and salt. Blend until creamy. Enjoy it warm.

D. Nourishing Bowls, Broths & Salad Boosters

46. Salmon & Roasted Veggie Salt Bowl

Ingredients:

- 1 salmon fillet
- 1 cup mixed vegetables (carrots, zucchini, bell peppers)
- 1 tablespoon olive oil

- 1/2 teaspoon pink salt
- Juice of ½ lemon

How to Make:
Preheat oven to 375°F (190°C). Toss veggies in oil and pink salt. Place on baking sheet with salmon. Roast for 20–25 minutes until fish flakes easily. Drizzle with lemon juice and serve warm in a bowl.

47. Sweet Potato Avocado Green Bowl

Ingredients:

- 1 small sweet potato (roasted or steamed)
- ½ avocado (sliced)
- 1 handful of arugula or spinach
- 1 teaspoon olive oil
- 1/4 teaspoon pink salt

How to Make:
Roast or steam sweet potato until soft. Layer into a bowl with greens and avocado. Drizzle with oil and sprinkle pink salt on top.

48. Warm Quinoa with Steamed Greens & Pink Salt

Ingredients:

- 1 cup cooked quinoa

- 1 cup steamed broccoli or kale
- 1/2 teaspoon pink salt
- Squeeze of lemon or apple cider vinegar

How to Make:
Cook quinoa and steam greens. Toss together in a bowl. Add pink salt and a splash of lemon juice. Mix well and enjoy warm.

49. Pink Salt Tahini Buddha Bowl

Ingredients:

- 1/2 cup cooked brown rice or quinoa
- 1/2 cup roasted chickpeas or tofu
- 1/2 cup raw or steamed veggies (carrot ribbons, spinach, cucumber)
- 1 tablespoon tahini
- 1/4 teaspoon pink salt

How to Make:
Arrange grains, protein, and veggies in a bowl. Mix tahini with a splash of warm water and pink salt to make a drizzle. Pour over the bowl before eating.

50. Salted Lentil Kale Nourish Bowl

Ingredients:

- 1/2 cup cooked lentils
- 1 cup sautéed kale
- 1/4 teaspoon turmeric
- 1/2 teaspoon pink salt
- 1 teaspoon olive oil

How to Make:
Sauté kale with turmeric and olive oil. Stir in cooked lentils and pink salt. Serve warm as a grounding, protein-rich bowl.

51. Sardine, Cucumber & Pink Salt Protein Bowl

Ingredients:

- 1 can sardines in olive oil
- ½ cucumber (sliced)
- ½ avocado
- 1/2 teaspoon pink salt
- Black pepper to taste

How to Make:
Arrange sardines, cucumber, and avocado in a bowl. Sprinkle pink salt and pepper. Eat chilled as a light, protein- and omega-3-rich lunch.

52. Salted Roasted Beet, Walnut & Arugula Salad

Ingredients:

- 1 small beet (roasted, chopped)
- 1 cup arugula
- 1 tablespoon chopped walnuts
- 1 tablespoon olive oil
- 1/4 teaspoon pink salt

How to Make:
Toss roasted beets, arugula, and walnuts in a bowl. Drizzle with olive oil and sprinkle with pink salt just before serving.

53. Golden Chickpea Protein Bowl with Salted Yogurt

Ingredients:

- 1/2 cup cooked chickpeas
- 1 teaspoon turmeric
- 1/2 cup plain Greek yogurt (or dairy-free alternative)
- 1/4 teaspoon pink salt
- A few fresh herbs (parsley or cilantro)

How to Make:
Warm chickpeas with turmeric. In a bowl, layer chickpeas and yogurt. Sprinkle with pink salt and herbs.

54. Steamed Broccoli, Hemp Seeds & Pink Salt Drizzle

Ingredients:

- 1 cup steamed broccoli
- 1 tablespoon hemp seeds
- 1/2 teaspoon pink salt
- 1 teaspoon lemon juice or olive oil

How to Make:
Steam broccoli until vibrant green. Top with hemp seeds and pink salt. Drizzle with lemon juice or olive oil before serving.

55. Avocado Egg Bowl with Seaweed & Salt

Ingredients:

- 2 boiled eggs
- ½ avocado
- 1 sheet nori (crumbled) or seaweed flakes
- 1/2 teaspoon pink salt

How to Make:
Slice eggs and avocado. Arrange in a bowl. Top with seaweed and pink salt. A high-protein, mineral-dense breakfast or lunch.

56. Lemon Salted Cabbage Slaw with Apple

Ingredients:

- 1 cup shredded cabbage
- 1/2 apple (thinly sliced)
- 1/2 teaspoon pink salt
- Juice of 1/2 lemon
- Optional: pinch of cumin or fennel seed

How to Make:
Massage cabbage with lemon juice and salt until slightly softened. Add apple and toss. Let it sit for 10 minutes before serving.

57. Brown Rice, Kimchi & Salted Egg Bowl

Ingredients:

- 1/2 cup cooked brown rice
- 1 boiled egg
- 1/4 cup kimchi
- 1/4 teaspoon pink salt
- Dash of sesame oil

How to Make:
Layer rice, sliced egg, and kimchi in a bowl. Sprinkle with pink salt and sesame oil. Eat warm or at room temperature.

58. Chopped Kale Tahini Salad with Pink Salt Crunch

Ingredients:

- 1 cup finely chopped kale
- 1 tablespoon tahini
- 1/2 teaspoon pink salt
- Juice of ½ lemon
- Optional: chopped almonds

How to Make:
Massage kale with lemon juice and salt. Let it sit for 5 minutes. Drizzle with tahini and toss. Add nuts for crunch if desired.

59. Roasted Carrot Wild Rice Bowl with Garlic Salt

Ingredients:

- 1/2 cup cooked wild rice
- 1 cup roasted carrots
- 1 clove garlic (roasted or minced)
- 1/2 teaspoon pink salt
- Drizzle of olive oil

How to Make:
Roast carrots with garlic and olive oil until tender. Serve over wild rice. Sprinkle with pink salt just before serving.

60. Rainbow Quinoa Bowl with Spiced Pink Salt Dressing

Ingredients:

- 1/2 cup cooked quinoa
- 1/2 cup chopped red bell pepper, cucumber, and purple cabbage
- 1/2 teaspoon pink salt
- 1 tablespoon olive oil
- 1/4 teaspoon cumin or smoked paprika

How to Make:
Combine quinoa and veggies in a bowl. Mix pink salt, oil, and spices in a cup to make dressing. Pour over bowl and toss.

E. Bloating Relief Teas, Mineral Snacks & PMS Soothers

61. Chamomile Pink Salt Calming Tea

Ingredients:

- 1 chamomile tea bag or 1 teaspoon dried chamomile
- 1 cup hot water
- Pinch of pink salt

- Optional: 1/2 teaspoon raw honey

How to Make:
Steep chamomile in hot water for 5–7 minutes. Stir in pink salt and honey if desired. Drink before bed or anytime stress rises.

62. Fennel-Ginger Bloat Relief Brew

Ingredients:

- 1/2 teaspoon fennel seeds
- 3 slices fresh ginger or 1/4 teaspoon grated ginger
- 1 cup water
- Pinch of pink salt

How to Make:
Boil fennel and ginger in water for 10 minutes. Strain and stir in pink salt. Sip warm tea to ease bloating after meals.

63. Salted Cacao Hormone Harmony Latte

Ingredients:

- 1 tablespoon raw cacao powder
- 1 cup almond or oat milk
- 1/4 teaspoon pink salt
- Optional: pinch of cinnamon or maca powder

How to Make:
Warm milk on the stove. Stir in cacao and pink salt until smooth. Add cinnamon or maca if using. Whisk well and drink slowly.

64. Lavender & Pink Salt Stress Ease Tea

Ingredients:

- 1 teaspoon dried lavender
- 1 cup hot water
- Pinch of pink salt
- Optional: lemon slice

How to Make:
Steep lavender in hot water for 5–10 minutes. Add pink salt and lemon if desired. Calming for both nerves and digestion.

65. Golden Milk with Pink Salt & Cinnamon

Ingredients:

- 1 cup almond or coconut milk
- 1/2 teaspoon turmeric
- 1/4 teaspoon cinnamon
- 1/8 teaspoon pink salt
- Optional: 1 teaspoon honey

How to Make:
Warm milk gently. Whisk in turmeric, cinnamon, and pink salt. Add honey if using. Drink before bed to support inflammation reduction and sleep.

66. PMS Soothing Raspberry Leaf Tea with Salt

Ingredients:

- 1 raspberry leaf tea bag
- 1 cup boiling water
- Pinch of pink salt
- Optional: a slice of fresh orange or lemon

How to Make:
Steep tea for 10 minutes. Stir in salt. Add a fruit slice if desired. Ideal during your cycle for cramp relief and hormone support.

67. Warm Lemon-Honey Pink Salt Tonic

Ingredients:

- 1 cup warm water
- Juice of ½ lemon
- 1 teaspoon raw honey
- Pinch of pink salt

How to Make:
Stir all ingredients into warm water until fully dissolved. Drink first thing in the morning or during low energy dips.

68. Pink Salted Pumpkin Seeds

Ingredients:

- 1/2 cup raw or roasted pumpkin seeds
- 1/4 teaspoon pink salt
- Optional: dash of smoked paprika or turmeric

How to Make:
Toss seeds with salt and optional seasoning. Eat as is or toast in a dry pan for 3–4 minutes for added crunch.

69. Salted Cucumber Bites with Hummus

Ingredients:

- 1 cucumber, sliced into rounds
- 1/2 cup hummus
- Pink salt to sprinkle

How to Make:
Arrange cucumber slices on a plate. Add a dollop of hummus on each. Sprinkle lightly with pink salt just before eating.

70. Roasted Pink Salt Chickpeas

Ingredients:

- 1 cup cooked chickpeas (canned or boiled)
- 1/2 teaspoon olive oil
- 1/2 teaspoon pink salt
- Optional: garlic powder, cumin, or paprika

How to Make:
Preheat oven to 400°F (200°C). Toss chickpeas in oil, salt, and spices. Roast for 25–30 minutes, shaking halfway. Cool before eating.

71. Baked Sweet Potato Fries with Paprika & Salt

Ingredients:

- 1 medium sweet potato (cut into wedges)
- 1 teaspoon olive oil
- 1/2 teaspoon pink salt
- 1/2 teaspoon smoked paprika

How to Make:
Preheat oven to 425°F (220°C). Toss sweet potato with oil and spices. Spread on a baking sheet. Bake for 30–35 minutes, flipping once.

72. Seaweed Snacks with Pink Salt & Sesame

Ingredients:

- 1 sheet nori or store-bought seaweed snacks
- Pink salt
- Optional: drizzle of toasted sesame oil or sesame seeds

How to Make:
Tear nori into pieces. Lightly brush with sesame oil (optional) and sprinkle pink salt on top. Eat it as a crunchy mineral snack.

73. Celery Almond Butter Pink Salt Snack

Ingredients:

- 2 celery stalks
- 1 tablespoon almond butter
- Pinch of pink salt

How to Make:
Cut celery into sticks. Fill each groove with almond butter. Sprinkle with salt for a crunchy, protein-rich snack.

74. Salted Avocado Half with Chili Flakes

Ingredients:

- 1 ripe avocado

- 1/2 teaspoon pink salt
- Pinch of chili flakes or paprika

How to Make:
Cut the avocado in half. Remove pit. Sprinkle salt and chili flakes directly onto the flesh. Eat with a spoon.

75. Apple Slices with Tahini & Sea Salt

Ingredients:

- 1 apple (sliced)
- 1 tablespoon tahini
- 1/4 teaspoon pink salt

How to Make:
Arrange apple slices on a plate. Drizzle tahini over each and sprinkle with salt. A perfect sweet-salty snack for hormone balance.

F. Pink Salt Mineral Water Tonics & Bedtime Calm Blends

76. Bedtime Pink Salt + Honey Tonic

Ingredients:

- 1 cup warm water
- 1/8 teaspoon pink salt
- 1 teaspoon raw honey

How to Make:
Stir salt and honey into warm water until fully dissolved. Sip slowly 30 minutes before bed to support adrenal recovery and overnight blood sugar balance.

77. Salted Chamomile Ginger Sleep Tea

Ingredients:

- 1 chamomile tea bag or 1 teaspoon dried chamomile
- 2 slices fresh ginger
- 1 cup boiling water
- Pinch of pink salt

How to Make:
Steep chamomile and ginger in boiling water for 7–10 minutes. Stir in pink salt and enjoy as a soothing nighttime tea.

78. Warm Cinnamon Milk with Pink Salt

Ingredients:

- 1 cup almond or oat milk
- 1/4 teaspoon ground cinnamon
- 1/8 teaspoon pink salt
- Optional: dash of vanilla extract

How to Make:
Warm milk gently. Whisk in cinnamon and pink salt. Add vanilla if using. Drink it warm and slow—it relaxes muscles and soothes digestion.

79. Magnesium Moon Milk with Pink Salt

Ingredients:

- 1 cup warm milk (dairy-free or dairy)
- 1/4 teaspoon magnesium powder (consult label)
- 1/8 teaspoon pink salt
- Pinch of nutmeg

How to Make:
Warm milk and whisk in magnesium, pink salt, and nutmeg. Sip in bed to support relaxation and deep sleep.

80. Calming Lemon-Balm Pink Salt Brew

Ingredients:

- 1 teaspoon dried lemon balm or 1 tea bag
- 1 cup hot water
- Pinch of pink salt
- Optional: 1 teaspoon honey

How to Make:
Steep lemon balm in hot water for 8–10 minutes. Stir in pink salt and honey if desired. Ideal for stress relief before sleep.

81. Hibiscus Rose Pink Salt Cooler

Ingredients:

- 1 hibiscus tea bag
- 1 teaspoon dried rose petals (optional)
- 1 cup hot water
- 1/8 teaspoon pink salt
- Ice (for serving cold)

How to Make:
Steep hibiscus and rose in hot water for 10 minutes. Strain and let cool. Add pink salt, pour over ice, and enjoy as a mineral-rich refreshment.

82. Salted Blueberry Herbal Water

Ingredients:

- 1/2 cup fresh or frozen blueberries
- 2 basil or mint leaves
- 1.5 cups water
- 1/8 teaspoon pink salt

- Optional: a squeeze of lemon

How to Make:
Muddle blueberries and herbs in the bottom of a jar. Add water and salt. Let it infuse for 5–10 minutes before sipping.

83. Turmeric Golden Moon Tonic

Ingredients:

- 1 cup almond or coconut milk
- 1/2 teaspoon turmeric powder
- Pinch of black pepper
- 1/8 teaspoon pink salt
- Optional: 1/2 teaspoon raw honey

How to Make:
Heat milk gently and whisk in turmeric, pepper, salt, and honey. This anti-inflammatory night drink relaxes muscles and eases pain.

84. Apple Cider Vinegar Sleep Elixir

Ingredients:

- 1 cup warm water
- 1 teaspoon apple cider vinegar
- 1/2 teaspoon raw honey
- 1/8 teaspoon pink salt

How to Make:
Stir all ingredients into warm water. Drink 30–60 minutes before bed to support digestion, blood sugar, and detox.

85. Salted Lavender Lemon Mocktail

Ingredients:

- 1/2 teaspoon dried lavender or 2 drops food-grade lavender essence
- 1 cup sparkling water
- Juice of 1/2 lemon
- Pinch of pink salt

How to Make:
Infuse lavender in warm water or add it directly with lemon and salt to sparkling water. Stir gently. Chill before sipping.

86. Warm Salted Almond-Coconut Drink

Ingredients:

- 1/2 cup almond milk
- 1/2 cup coconut milk
- 1/8 teaspoon pink salt
- Optional: dash of cinnamon or cardamom

How to Make:
Warm the almond and coconut milk together. Stir in pink salt and optional spices. Drink in the evening to replenish minerals and soothe cravings.

87. Salt + Collagen Hot Chocolate

Ingredients:

- 1 tablespoon cacao or cocoa powder
- 1 cup warm milk (any kind)
- 1 scoop collagen powder
- 1/8 teaspoon pink salt
- Optional: touch of maple syrup

How to Make:
Whisk all ingredients together in warm milk until smooth. Drink before bed for skin support, joint recovery, and deep sleep.

88. Salted Licorice Root Nerve Tonic

Ingredients:

- 1 teaspoon dried licorice root (or 1 tea bag)
- 1 cup water
- 1/8 teaspoon pink salt

How to Make:
Simmer licorice root in water for 10 minutes, strain, and add pink salt. Great for adrenal and nervous system support.

89. Mineral Water with Fresh Mint + Grapefruit

Ingredients:

- 1 cup mineral or filtered water
- 2 slices fresh grapefruit
- 3 mint leaves
- 1/8 teaspoon pink salt

How to Make:
Muddle grapefruit and mint in the bottom of a glass. Add water and pink salt. Let it sit for 2–3 minutes before sipping.

90. Salted Rooibos Vanilla Sleep Tea

Ingredients:

- 1 rooibos tea bag
- 1 cup boiling water
- 1/8 teaspoon pink salt
- Optional: splash of vanilla extract or plant milk

How to Make:
Steep rooibos in boiling water for 7–10 minutes. Add pink salt and

optional vanilla. Drink warm milk before bed to promote deep, restful sleep.

G. Hormonal, Thyroid & Adrenal-Supportive Salt Blends

91. Morning Mineral Blend (Pink Salt, Lemon Peel, Ginger Powder)

Ingredients:

- 2 tablespoons pink salt
- 1 tablespoon finely grated lemon zest (dried or fresh)
- 1 teaspoon ground ginger

How to Make:
Mix all ingredients thoroughly and store in a small jar. Add a pinch to your morning lemon water or warm water ritual. Supports digestion, adrenal wake-up, and liver function.

92. Hormone Harmony Sprinkle (Seaweed, Pink Salt, Nettle Leaf)

Ingredients:

- 2 tablespoons pink salt
- 1 tablespoon powdered seaweed (kelp or dulse)
- 1 tablespoon dried nettle leaf (finely ground)

How to Make:
Combine well and store airtight. Sprinkle over cooked vegetables, eggs, or into soups. Rich in iodine and minerals to support thyroid health and estrogen balance.

93. Adrenal Calm Salt Mix (Lavender, Cardamom, Pink Salt)

Ingredients:

- 2 tablespoons pink salt
- 1 teaspoon dried culinary lavender (finely ground)
- 1/2 teaspoon ground cardamom

How to Make:
Stir ingredients together and store sealed. Use a small pinch in warm tea or milk in the evening. This blend soothes adrenal glands and promotes nervous system relaxation.

94. Energy Boost Sprinkle (Cayenne, Pink Salt, Lemon Zest)

Ingredients:

- 2 tablespoons pink salt
- 1/2 teaspoon cayenne pepper
- 1 teaspoon dried lemon zest or powder

How to Make:
Mix and keep in a spice jar. Add a pinch to your morning water or a savory bowl. This blend stimulates circulation, boosts metabolism, and supports fat burning.

95. Gut Health Blend (Fennel Seed, Turmeric, Pink Salt)

Ingredients:

- 1 tablespoon ground fennel seed
- 1 tablespoon ground turmeric
- 2 tablespoons pink salt
- Pinch of black pepper (optional)

How to Make:
Stir together and store dry. Add a pinch to warm water before meals or use in lentil stews or roasted vegetables. Supports digestion, liver detox, and reduces bloating.

96. Sleep Salt Mix (Chamomile, Nutmeg, Pink Salt)

Ingredients:

- 2 tablespoons pink salt
- 1 teaspoon dried chamomile flowers (finely ground)
- 1/2 teaspoon nutmeg powder

How to Make:
Blend well and store in a cool, dark place. Add a pinch to warm bedtime drinks or honey water. This blend encourages relaxation and deeper sleep.

97. Craving Killer Mix (Cinnamon, Ginger, Pink Salt)

Ingredients:

- 1 tablespoon cinnamon powder
- 1 tablespoon ground ginger
- 2 tablespoons pink salt

How to Make:
Mix and seal in a glass jar. Add to smoothies, teas, or sprinkle on apple slices or warm oatmeal. Balances blood sugar and reduces sugar cravings.

98. Detox Day Blend (Dandelion, Pink Salt, ACV Powder)

Ingredients:

- 1 tablespoon dandelion leaf powder
- 1/2 tablespoon apple cider vinegar powder (optional)
- 2 tablespoons pink salt

How to Make:
Stir well and store dry. Use 1/4 teaspoon in water or broth on detox days. Helps flush the liver and support gentle daily cleansing.

99. Lymphatic Support Salt Mix (Lemon Balm, Pink Salt, Parsley)

Ingredients:

- 1 tablespoon dried lemon balm (ground)
- 1 tablespoon dried parsley (finely ground)
- 2 tablespoons pink salt

How to Make:
Mix and keep in an airtight jar. Use in broths, soups, or warm teas. This blend helps stimulate lymphatic flow and reduce puffiness.

100. PMS Ease Blend (Rose, Raspberry Leaf, Pink Salt)

Ingredients:

- 1 teaspoon dried rose petals (crushed)
- 1 tablespoon raspberry leaf (ground)
- 2 tablespoons pink salt

How to Make:
Combine and mix well. Stir a pinch into warm tea or honey water during your cycle. Helps ease cramps, soothe mood swings, and replenish minerals lost during menstruation.

101. General Wellness Salt Blend (Turmeric, Black Pepper, Pink Salt)

Ingredients:

- 2 tablespoons pink salt
- 1 tablespoon turmeric powder
- 1/4 teaspoon black pepper

How to Make:
Mix and store dry. Use daily in warm drinks, on roasted veggies, or in broths. Anti-inflammatory, immune-supporting, and ideal for daily mineral maintenance.

How to Use These Blends

Each of these salt blends can be added to

- Warm water or herbal tea
- Smoothies and tonics
- Soups, stews, and broths
- Cooked grains or sautéed veggies
- Sprinkled lightly on protein dishes

Just 1/8 to 1/4 teaspoon daily can shift your mineral balance, calm your system, and support metabolism, mood, digestion, and hormones—without pills or perfection.

This is how you reclaim healing with what's already in your kitchen.

Chapter 9

BEYOND THE SCALE – ENERGY, SLEEP & MOOD TRANSFORMATION

There's a moment in every woman's wellness journey when she realizes the goal was never really the number on the scale. Not truly. What she's been craving—what she's always been chasing—was how she thought that number would make her feel.

Light. Clear. Energized. Rested. Radiant. Free.

Weight loss is often the doorway. But the destination? It's something far deeper.

This is the hidden magic of the Pink Salt Ritual: it's not just about burning fat—it's about lighting up your life. And when done consistently, with intention, it doesn't just shape your body. It transforms your *being.*

In this chapter, we step past the numbers and dig into the subtle but powerful shifts that thousands of women have reported: glowing skin, deeper sleep, fewer mood crashes, restored energy, and a renewed emotional balance that no "weight loss plan" has ever offered them.

The Real Wins: What Readers Report First

Ask any woman who's faithfully done the Pink Salt Morning Ritual for three weeks or more, and her story almost always begins the same way:

> "I didn't expect to feel this good—this *quickly*."

Before the inches drop or the pants fit looser, it starts with something softer. She wakes up less groggy. Her mood feels steadier. She doesn't crash mid-afternoon like before. And she finds herself smiling... for no reason.

That's when it clicks.

This isn't a diet. It's a *daily homecoming*—a gentle reset for the systems that have long been ignored in the noise of calorie-counting and scale-obsessing.

Skin That Glows From Within

When your cells are hydrated with the right minerals—not just plain water—you begin to glow. Literally.

Pink salt carries over 80 trace minerals, including zinc, magnesium, calcium, and potassium—nutrients that skin *drinks* in to rebuild its natural radiance. These minerals play a direct role in collagen production, skin barrier protection, and pH balance.

But the magic is in the internal shift:

- **Reduced puffiness** from lower water retention

- **Improved circulation** from boosted electrolyte balance
- **Balanced oil production** from stabilized hormones

Instead of chasing beauty through serums and scrubs, the ritual turns beauty into a *byproduct* of inner balance.

Salt & Circadian Rhythm—The Natural Sleep Reset

Most women don't have a "weight problem." They have a **rest problem.**

Chronic sleep deprivation and hormonal burnout keep cortisol high, blood sugar erratic, and fat locked in place. And the harder they try—more fasting, more cardio, more stress—the worse it gets.

But here's what the pink salt trick does quietly, every morning:

It signals your body that the day has begun. It anchors your **circadian rhythm.**

The blend of minerals—especially magnesium and sodium—works as an internal clock cue, nudging your adrenal system to regulate wake-up and wind-down cycles. Over time, women report:

- Falling asleep faster
- Waking up without alarm fatigue
- No more 3 a.m. anxiety spikes
- Dreams returning
- Feeling *rested*, not just unconscious

Some even replace melatonin with a pinch of pink salt in warm herbal tea before bed—supporting natural melatonin production without dependency.

Mood, Mind & the Gut-Brain Connection

It's hard to feel light in your body when your mind is foggy, anxious, or low.

That's where pink salt shows up again—not as a sedative, but as a *signal booster* between your gut and brain.

Your digestive system is home to over 90% of your body's serotonin receptors. That means how your gut feels, digests, and detoxes directly impacts your emotions.

Here's how pink salt helps:

- It boosts **stomach acid**, improving nutrient absorption
- It aids **bile production**, helping the liver clear excess estrogen
- It **replenishes electrolytes**, which regulate neuron firing and mental clarity
- It supports the **vagus nerve**, your brain-gut communication superhighway

The result? Fewer mood swings. Less emotional eating. More presence. More peace.

Women say they no longer feel like they're "fighting themselves" after a stressful day. They just drink their ritual… and feel *recentered*.

Why You Crash Less and Do More (Without Forcing It)

Imagine this: You go through a full day, handle work, make decisions, deal with your family, and still have enough energy left to move your body—not out of guilt, but *because you want to.*

This is what happens when your blood sugar stops spiking and crashing.

The trace minerals in pink salt (particularly magnesium and potassium) stabilize glucose uptake at the cellular level. That means fewer sugar dips, fewer mid-morning hangries, and less of that drained, can't-keep-my-eyes-open-at-3pm feeling.

Women report:

- Greater stamina through workouts or busy days
- Less caffeine dependency
- Fewer sugar cravings in the afternoon
- Improved productivity and focus
- Even libido returns as adrenal stress fades

The Salt + Sun + Soul Synergy

In ancient wellness systems, healing was always holistic. You didn't just treat symptoms—you nourished the body, mind, and *spirit* in rhythm with nature.

That's exactly what this ritual revives.

Many women begin their pink salt drink by a window, in sunlight, in stillness. Just 5 minutes. That moment, repeated, becomes sacred.

Here's what that small act gives you:

- **Salt** replenishes your minerals, restoring your internal power grid
- **Sun** resets your circadian rhythm and charges your vitamin D stores
- **Stillness** recalibrates your nervous system, lowering cortisol

It becomes a ritual of **sovereignty**—a time where the world doesn't own you yet.

You reclaim your energy. Your clarity. Your center.

And that, more than weight loss, is what keeps women coming back.

What Happens After the 21 Days?

After three weeks of consistent practice, most women don't want to stop—not because they're trying to stay "on plan," but because they *feel like themselves* again.

They report:

- No more snoozing alarms
- Stable moods during PMS
- Clearer skin, reduced breakouts

- Regular digestion without bloat
- Emotional eating episodes fading
- Better boundaries and calmer responses
- A quiet joy in their mornings

This isn't about perfection. It's about **permission**—to feel good without punishment, without restriction, and without fear of "messing it up."

It's a feeling you can build your life on.

Closing Thought: You Were Never Meant to Chase Energy

You were meant to *carry it.*

Not the jittery kind that burns out by noon. But the deep, humming current of vitality that flows when your body is supported, your mind is nourished, and your soul is at peace.

That's what the pink salt trick offers—not a miracle, but a return.

To rhythm. To radiance. To your real self.

And that, dear reader, is the transformation that no diet in the world has ever delivered.

Let's keep going.

Chapter 10

How to Ditch the Pills, Diets, and Start Over Naturally

There comes a moment—quiet but undeniable—when you finally look at the lineup of powders, pills, calorie apps, and half-finished health fads on your shelf… and ask:

"Why am I still not well?"

You've done what they told you: the fasting, the green capsules, the low-carb panic, the motivational mantras. And yet, somewhere beneath all of it, your body is still begging—**not for more effort**, but for something simpler. Something real.

This chapter is your permission slip to stop chasing artificial fixes—and start over naturally.

Because the truth is this: **your body already knows how to heal.** It just needs the noise to stop, and the support to begin.

Let's break the cycle.

The Myth of More: Why Modern Wellness Leaves You Exhausted

Walk down any health aisle or scroll through #WellnessTok, and it's easy to believe that "health" is a product you haven't bought yet.

A supplement you're missing.

A protocol you haven't cracked.

But real wellness doesn't live in a bottle—it lives in your **rhythm.**

Pills may promise instant fixes, but they rarely address the deep fatigue, the hormone chaos, the nervous system overload, or the mineral depletion that most women silently carry.

The more you chase "solutions," the more fragmented you feel.

The Pink Salt Ritual, by contrast, asks only this:

> Wake up. Breathe. Drink deeply from the earth.
> Support your cells. Ground your body. Repeat.

That's it. No exotic ingredients. No overnight shipping. No dependency.

It's not just simplicity—it's sovereignty.

Why Pink Salt Replaces 5+ Products You Don't Actually Need

Let's look at what pink salt, used intentionally, gently replaces:

1. Electrolyte Supplements

Most electrolyte powders are loaded with artificial sweeteners, food dyes, and cheap minerals that flush out as fast as they enter.

Pink salt delivers sodium, magnesium, potassium, calcium, and trace minerals in a naturally balanced form your body *recognizes and absorbs*. It actually stays where it's needed—inside your cells.

2. Magnesium Capsules

Magnesium is essential for sleep, digestion, hormone balance, and over 300 enzymatic functions. Instead of relying on hard-to-absorb synthetic forms, pink salt contains magnesium in a bioavailable, micro-dosed format—gentle, daily, and cumulative.

3. Digestive Enzymes

If your stomach acid is low (common in stressed-out women), your digestion is likely poor—even if you're eating "clean." Pink salt boosts hydrochloric acid production naturally, helping your body extract nutrients and reduce bloating without pills.

4. Hormone Support Stacks

Cortisol, insulin, and leptin—the big three weight-regulating hormones—don't need a supplement cocktail. They need rhythm, nourishment, and calm. Pink salt helps regulate blood sugar, calm the adrenals, and re-sensitize your body's hunger cues—all key to hormonal recalibration.

5. Energy Powders & Focus Boosters

Feeling tired isn't always a caffeine problem. It's often a mineral problem. The right salt helps your mitochondria (cellular energy factories) fire properly. No crash. No jitters. Just real, sustainable energy.

When you support your system at the *root*, you realize how many products you never needed in the first place.

Debunking the Myths: Salt, Iodine & Blood Pressure

Let's be clear: the fear around salt is **not** about pink Himalayan salt. It's about *refined, industrial salt*—the white table kind stripped of all minerals and laced with anti-caking agents and chemicals.

Here's the truth behind the myths:

MYTH 1: Salt causes high blood pressure.

REALITY: Refined table salt may contribute to hypertension in *some* individuals. But **mineral-rich natural salts** like Himalayan pink salt often help regulate blood pressure by supporting hydration and adrenal function.

MYTH 2: Salt leads to water retention.

REALITY: Water retention is often caused by **mineral imbalance**—not salt excess. Paradoxically, the right kind of salt (with magnesium and potassium) can *help you release excess water* by restoring cellular osmosis.

MYTH 3: You'll become iodine deficient.

REALITY: Iodine is important—but your body only needs **trace** amounts. You can get iodine from sea vegetables, seafood, or small doses of iodized salt if necessary. Pink salt isn't an iodine *supplement*, but it doesn't *deplete* iodine either.

You are not fragile. You are not a statistic. And you're allowed to learn what *actually* works for your unique body.

Reading Labels: The "Salt Hacks" You Should Actually Avoid

Not all pink salts are created equal—and not all wellness products with "salt" on the label are trustworthy. Here's what to be cautious about:

- **Flavored electrolyte mixes:** Many are packed with sucralose, dyes, or maltodextrin (a sugar spike in disguise).
- **Pink salt sprays or mists:** Marketed for beauty but often overpriced and ineffective compared to drinking it.
- **Salt pills in plastic capsules:** Your body digests real salt better as a *dissolved mineral*, not a powder in a capsule.

Instead, choose **pure, unrefined, hand-mined pink Himalayan salt**—free of additives, moisture-proofed agents, or bleaching.

Simple. Transparent. Authentic.

Pink Salt Pills vs. The Ritual: What's the Difference?

You might wonder: if pink salt is so powerful, can I just take a capsule and skip the ritual?

The answer: **you'd miss the magic.**

Yes, technically you could get *some* mineral benefit from salt pills—but you'd miss:

- The **hydration synergy** of warm water + minerals
- The **nervous system reset** of sipping slowly in stillness
- The **gut-brain signaling** from the taste of salt on your tongue
- The **habit stack** of starting your day with presence and intention

This isn't about supplements. It's about *ceremony.*

A pink salt drink is more than chemistry—it's a **moment of reconnection.**

You can't bottle that. But you can choose it—every single day.

Starting Over: One Mineral at a Time

Maybe you've been burned by every diet. Maybe your cabinet is full of supplements that promised glow and gave you nothing. Maybe you're tired of feeling like your body is a problem to fix.

This is your invitation:

> Tolet it be easy.
> To let it be daily.
> To let it be *yours*.

Start with one small ritual: the Pink Salt Drink.

Let it root you each morning.

Let it remind you of your natural rhythm.

Then build from there:

- Add sunlight.
- Add breath.
- Add nourishment, not restriction.
- Add movement that brings joy, not punishment.

And slowly, your lifestyle becomes a healing ecosystem—crafted from *care*, not control.

Final Words: You Were Never Broken—Just Overwhelmed

Wellness has been overcomplicated by people trying to sell you a "fix."

But your body doesn't need fixing. It needs *remembering*.

It needs minerals. Sleep. Joy. Rhythm. Safety. Stillness. And a little salt.

Start there.

Ditch the pills.

Release the rigid plans.

Choose the ritual.

And let this be the chapter where everything begins again—only softer, simpler, and more soulfully than ever before.

Chapter 11

FREQUENTLY ASKED QUESTIONS & REAL-WORLD SUCCESS STORIES

Somewhere between your first sip of warm pink salt water and your third week of glowing skin, fewer cravings, and better sleep—you start asking different questions.

Not "Is this working?"
But: **"Why didn't I know about this sooner?"**

This chapter is for the real-life stories, quiet wins, tearful breakthroughs, and everything women have asked as they stepped into this radically gentle reset.

Whether you're just getting started or deep into your transformation, consider this your Pink Salt Sisterhood's collective wisdom.

What if I miss a day?

Don't worry. This is **not** a diet or a punishment-based plan. Your body doesn't need you to be perfect—it needs consistency and compassion.

If you miss a day:

- Simply resume the next morning.
- Don't "double up" or overcompensate.
- Trust that your body is resilient—and your healing doesn't unravel from one pause.

Remember: healing happens in rhythm, not in streaks. Let your nervous system *relax into progress.*

Is it safe for high blood pressure or thyroid conditions?

This is one of the most common (and understandable) concerns. Let's unpack it carefully.

Blood Pressure

Most conventional doctors are trained to warn against "salt" due to its association with **refined table salt**, which **lacks minerals** and causes imbalance in some individuals.

But **unrefined pink Himalayan salt** contains **over 80 trace minerals**, which actually support

- Improved hydration (reducing blood volume stress)
- Calmer adrenal function (reducing cortisol spikes)
- Better potassium-sodium balance (supporting vascular tone)

That said, if you have a **known salt-sensitive condition**, it's wise to:

- Use ¼ tsp or less in your morning drink
- Monitor your response carefully
- Speak with a functional or integrative practitioner familiar with natural mineral therapy

Thyroid Health

Iodine is essential for thyroid hormone production. While pink salt does not contain added iodine (unlike iodized table salt), most people can obtain iodine from:

- Seaweed (e.g., nori, dulse, kelp)
- Seafood
- Eggs and dairy (if consumed)

You can combine pink salt with iodine-rich foods in your diet. Pink salt *does not interfere* with thyroid function. In fact, its mineral profile may reduce the **adrenal-thyroid burden** by helping regulate cortisol.

As always, personalized medicine > generalized fear.

What kind of salt should I use (and avoid)?

This is crucial. Not all pink salts are equal—and not all salts are even real.

Best Choices:

- **Pure Himalayan pink salt** (hand-mined, fine or coarse ground)
- **Celtic sea salt** (grayish tone, wet or moist)
- **Redmond Real Salt** (mined in Utah, trace minerals intact)

Avoid:

- Refined table salt (bleached, stripped, and chemically treated)
- "Pink salt" blends with additives or anti-caking agents
- Fluorescent white salts labeled "sea salt" with no trace minerals

Always check that your salt is

- **Additive-free**
- **Non-irradiated**
- **Responsibly sourced**

Real salt has **color, texture, and life** in it. It feels like food from the earth—because it is.

How long until I see results?

The short answer: *It depends on your body's current state, history, and stress load.*

But here's what we've seen from thousands of women:

- **Day 1–3:** Less brain fog, easier morning energy, reduced sugar cravings
- **Day 4–7:** Better bowel movements, subtle mood improvements, less bloating
- **Day 8–14:** More stable hunger cues, clearer skin, deeper sleep
- **Day 15–21:** Reduced PMS symptoms, weight shifts (water loss + fat mobilization), restored confidence

This isn't magic. It's **mineral repletion**—and your body *loves* to work well once supported.

That said, **don't chase symptoms—track rhythms.** Even if weight loss is slow, better sleep, less snacking, improved mood, and hormone balance are *worth their weight in gold.*

Real Stories, Real Women, Real Wins

The following voices are not celebrities or influencers—they're women like you.

They didn't need willpower. They just needed a fresh rhythm—and a little salt.

Fatima, 42—Nurse, Mom of 3

"I used to wake up dreading the day. Coffee didn't touch my fatigue. But after 5 days of the morning pink salt drink, I wasn't crashing at 2pm. I

stopped needing afternoon sugar just to function. And I've lost 9 pounds without thinking about it."

Sarah, 29—Freelancer with PCOS

"I've tried keto, IF, veganism—you name it. All made me feel crazy around food. This pink salt ritual stabilized my hunger in a way nothing else did. I went from binge-eating chips at night to not even thinking about snacks. My acne cleared too!"

Monica, 56—Perimenopausal Queen

"My belly just wouldn't budge. I thought it was age. Turns out, it was water retention and stress. Within 3 weeks of starting, I felt lighter, even before I saw weight change. My face depuffed. My rings fit again. And the night sweats? Gone."

Aramide, 35—Entrepreneur in Lagos

"I travel a lot and live in chaos. I used to skip meals, then overeat. This one habit gave me grounding. The calm I feel after my morning drink... it's sacred. I'm no longer tempted by crazy detox teas. This is the first time I trust my body."

Vivian, 63—Retired Teacher

"I thought I was too old to lose weight naturally. I was on thyroid meds and still gaining. But after a month on the salt ritual, I've lost 7 pounds, my bloating is 90% gone, and I feel sharp again. I'm telling every woman over 50 I know."

Reader-Reported Benefits: The Unexpected Wins

While the ritual is known for weight loss and energy, here are some **less obvious but frequently reported results:**

- **Better mood regulation** during PMS and hormonal swings
- **Less puffiness in face and joints**
- **Improved digestion and less gas after meals**
- **Fewer cravings at night** (especially for sugar or carbs)
- **Deeper sleep** without needing melatonin
- **Improved bowel regularity** and less constipation
- **Easier morning wake-ups** (without an alarm)
- **Less anxiety and heart palpitations**
- **More motivation to walk, stretch, and move** daily

One reader said it best:

> "This doesn't just reset your metabolism—it resets your **relationship** with your body.

If You're Reading This, You're Already Winning

Whether you've lost 15 pounds, broken your sugar addiction, or simply remembered what calm feels like—you've done something powerful:

You said no to complexity.
You said no to shame.
You said yes to something beautifully simple.

That's radical.

That's healing.

That's what this movement is about.

So wherever you are in your journey—whether it's your first pink drink or your 90th—know this:

You're part of something bigger.

And it's only the beginning.

Chapter 12

Stay Light, Stay Balanced—Your Long-Term Ritual Blueprint

It starts with a pinch of salt.

That one intentional act—a glass of mineralized water in the morning—becomes more than just hydration. It becomes a promise. A reset. A sacred yes to your well-being, before the noise of the world has a chance to pull you away from yourself.

This final chapter is not about rules or strict plans. It's about remembering what your body already knows. Your body craves rhythm. It thrives in simplicity. It repairs itself when supported, not micromanaged.

You have the tools now. Let's build your long-term blueprint.

Your Metabolism: A Daily Relationship, Not a Crisis

Most women have been taught to treat their metabolism like a malfunctioning machine—something to fix when it's broken, punish when it's slow, and fear when it stalls. But what if we stop fighting it? What if we treat it like a relationship instead?

Your metabolism is not your enemy. It is your body's whisper, asking for rhythm, nourishment, and safety. The Pink Salt Ritual is just the first spark. Sustaining your lightness and balance comes from staying in dialogue with your body each day.

Your metabolism listens when you:

- Start your morning with mineral-rich hydration.
- Give it gentle movement, not punishment.
- Respect hunger and fullness cues.
- Prioritize rest, not restriction.

It's not about never eating late again or always getting 10,000 steps. It's about noticing how your body feels when you honor it.

The 90-Day Lifestyle Rhythm

If you've completed the 21-Day Pink Salt Metabolic Reset Plan, you've already built the foundation. Now, we shift from a reset to a rhythm.

Here's how to structure your next 90 days with flow:

Months 1–3: Build, Balance, Integrate

- **Month 1 – Deepen the Ritual:** Focus on consistency. Continue your morning pink salt drink. Track how different versions (with lemon, ginger, etc.) make you feel. Observe your digestion, cravings, and mood.
- **Month 2—Layer the Lifestyle: Start** integrating other

pink salt recipes from Chapter 8 into your meals. Choose one meal daily to anchor with a pink salt-based preparation. Practice gratitude and hydration together as a micro-morning ritual.

- **Month 3 – Flow into Freedom: This** is where rituals become identity. You don't force the habit—you crave it. You'll start instinctively knowing when your body needs minerals, when to rest, and when to move. Let yourself evolve from routine into intuitive living.

Micro-Habits That Keep You Light

Small things create massive shifts when repeated daily.

1. **Salt-First Mornings:** Before screens, before stress—drink your salt blend.

2. **Gratitude Glass:** While sipping, name 3 things you love about your body.

3. **Mineral Moments:** Add pink salt to one drink or meal per day consciously.

4. **Sodium-Supported Sleep:** Try your bedtime salt blend from Chapter 8.

5. **Bloat Check-Ins:** When you feel puffy, hydrate with lemon + salt water.

6. **Joyful Movement:** Walk, stretch, dance. No rules. Just movement that feels good.

These habits are light. Sustainable. They don't require a gym, app, or accountability partner. Just you, your body, and some minerals.

What to Do When You Fall Off Track

Here's the truth: you will.

You'll skip a ritual. You'll eat late and wake up foggy. You'll forget your salt drink, or you'll have a week of travel and disruption.

But here's the deeper truth: you don't start over. You return.

You return to your breath. You return to your water. You return to your salt.

And when you do, your body remembers. It doesn't hold grudges. It holds wisdom.

There is no wagon to fall off of. There is only the present moment and the next healing choice you can make.

Ritual + Rhythm = Resilience

The women who succeed long term aren't perfect. They're not always disciplined. But they are anchored in ritual. They've replaced willpower with rhythm. They've traded restriction for replenishment. They no longer wait to feel broken before they give themselves care.

Pink salt becomes a physical symbol of that care.

A sprinkle in your soup. A pinch in your morning drink. A jar by your bedside.

It whispers, "You don't need to hustle to heal." You just need to return. Again and again.

Write Your Ritual Blueprint

Before you close this chapter, take five minutes. Journal your own.

- What version of the pink salt morning ritual will you commit to?
- Which 2–3 salt recipes from Chapter 8 feel realistic to integrate weekly?
- What movement do you want to explore that feels joyful?
- What does lightness feel like in your body, not just your weight?
- What support do you need (space, silence, encouragement, tools) to stay balanced?

Your Opinion Matters!

Thank You for Reading!

Dear Reader,

Thank you for taking the time to read my work. Sharing resourceful information and ideas with readers like you is one of the greatest joys of being an author.

If you found this book valuable, entertaining, or thought-provoking—or even if you have suggestions for improvement—I'd greatly appreciate your honest feedback in a review. Your thoughts not only help me grow but also guide other readers in discovering books they might enjoy or find useful.

Leaving a review is simple, and it makes a big difference. Thank you for your support—it truly means a lot!

With gratitude!

Jerry A. Hannon

About the Author

Jerry A. Hannon is a passionate wellness researcher, culinary innovator, and advocate for sustainable, non-restrictive approaches to health and weight loss. With over a decade of exploration into ancient healing traditions, mineral therapy, and nutritional ritualism, Jerry has dedicated his life to helping others reclaim their vitality—one intentional morning at a time.

Frustrated by the revolving door of diets, pills, and fads that left real people feeling defeated, Jerry began digging deeper. What he found was a simple truth: the body doesn't thrive under punishment—it heals under rhythm, nourishment, and mineral balance. His groundbreaking work on the *pink salt trick* has since sparked a global reset for thousands of readers, empowering women and men to transform their health without fear, restriction, or starvation.

When he's not writing or speaking, Jerry can be found creating mineral-rich recipes, walking barefoot in nature, and helping people reconnect with their intuition through food and mindful living.

Jerry A. Hannon is not just teaching wellness—he's living proof that healing begins with simplicity.

Made in the USA
Middletown, DE
04 November [illegible]

Made in the USA
Monee, IL
04 November 2026

67391584R10085